The New Consultation

Developing doctor–patient communication

David Pendleton
Theo Schofield
Peter Tate
Peter Havelock

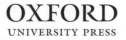

OXFORD
UNIVERSITY PRESS

OXFORD

UNIVERSITY PRESS

Great Clarendon Street, Oxford OX2 6DP

Oxford University Press is a department of the University of Oxford.
It furthers the University's objective of excellence in research, scholarship,
and education by publishing worldwide in

Oxford New York

Auckland Bangkok Buenos Aires Cape Town Chennai
Dar es Salaam Delhi Hong Kong Istanbul Karachi Kolkata
Kuala Lumpur Madrid Melbourne Mexico City Mumbai Nairobi
São Paulo Shanghai Taipei Tokyo Toronto

Oxford is a registered trade mark of Oxford University Press
in the UK and in certain other countries

Published in the United States
by Oxford University Press Inc., New York

A catalogue record for this title is available from the British Library

Library of Congress Cataloging in Publication Data
(Data available)
ISBN 0 19 263288 4

10 9 8 7 6 5 4 3 2 1

Typeset by Newgen Imaging Systems (P) Ltd., Chennai, India
Printed in Great Britain
on acid-free paper by
T. J. International Ltd, Padstow

For Reflexion

If I want to succeed
To bring a man towards a certain goal
I have to start finding out where he is
And start just there

The one who cannot do that
Fools himself
When he thinks he can help others

To be able to help someone
I certainly have to know more
But first of all
I have to know what he understands

If I can't do that
It will not help that I can and know more

If I still want to show how much I can
It is because I am vain and arrogant
And actually want to be admired of the other
Instead of helping him

All genuine helpfulness
Starts with being humble before the one I want to help
And I have to understand
That helping
Is not wanting to master
But to serve
If I can't do that
I am incapable of helping anyone

Sören Kirkegaard 1813–1855 translated by Dr Cecilia Ryding 2002

Contents

1 Introduction

The consultation: an approach to learning and teaching was published by Oxford University Press in 1984 (Pendleton *et al.* 1984). It was the forerunner of this volume. Our approach had two principal ingredients. The first was a model of an effective consultation in which doctor and patient work together to define problems and decide how they should be managed. The second was a method of teaching in which teacher and learner discover how to build on the learner's strengths to enhance his or her effectiveness.

There are a number of parallels between these processes. We described a style of consulting with patients in which the central purpose was to identify and to meet the patient's needs: a patient centred style of consulting. We also described a style of teaching in which learners were encouraged to identify their own strengths and weakness and to set the agenda for their teaching: a learner centred style of teaching. We described the consultation as part of a 'cycle of care' in which patients' understanding and ability to manage their own health are enhanced at each consultation. We continue to believe that the central purpose of teaching is to help our learners obtain greater understanding of their own consulting style and the ways in which they can develop and become more effective.

This introduction is, in part, a brief link between our first and the current book. Our original work was the result of collaboration between a social psychologist who was conducting research in doctor–patient communication, and three general practitioners involved in vocational training (VT) for general practice. The authors' backgrounds spanned teaching, research, psychology, interest in anthropology, Balint training, and practical experience of consulting with patients. These were brought together in our approach to the consultation.

In preparing the current volume, we discussed whether, after nearly two decades, we had to make small amendments and additions—to produce a second edition—or whether the book had to be completely re-written. Our consensus was that much of the writing needed to be new that the literature needed to be newly reviewed, and that much needed to be revisited. In these pages you will find a mix of updated concepts that arise from our more recent experiences and new research, but many of the propositions in the original book remain.

In preparing this volume we have attempted to remain focused on a particular readership. Essentially we are writing for practitioners and their teachers, rather than for researchers or academics. For this reason, we are not attempting to be comprehensive or encyclopaedic in our coverage of the issues or the relevant literature, but illustrative. We are adopting the position of generalists interpreting the literature through the eyes of our own experience.

The cycle of care

In the first book we described the *cycle of care* as a way to organize and understand the available evidence about the process of care in which the consultation plays a central part. The cycle describes the sequence of events around the consultation and how the various factors modify each other. It describes the antecedents of the consultation—those events that happen to people before they come to the doctor—and the immediate, intermediate,and long-term outcomes of the consultation. The cycle as a whole describes the central importance of the patients' understanding in influencing how they approach the consultation, how they behave during the consultation, and the actions they take after the consultation. The cycle indicates to doctors how effective consulting might be achieved, and how subsequent consultations can be influenced by enhancing patients' health understanding in *each* consultation. Chapter 2 describes the model more fully.

Throughout the first volume, there was mention of some of the ethical issues around the consultation and other contextual issues. Over the intervening years these issues have become more complex, and yet in some ways clearer, as a result of the many developments in thinking on patient-centredness and on patients' autonomy. These issues are discussed more fully in Chapter 3. Understanding the patient, what they bring to the consultation, and what the outcomes may be is discussed in Chapter 4.

The cycle of care describes the antecedents and consequences of each consultation for the doctor as well as the patient. It also highlights the societal and professional contexts in which he or she works. All these issues are further developed and discussed in Chapter 5.

The tasks of the consultation

Once we had described the cycle of care it was not difficult to define the contents of an effective consultation that would make the cycle of care work for the patient and encourage health improvement. In the first book we introduced *tasks* for the consultation as a clear statement of the consultation's purpose. Tasks were also seen to be the ideal starting point for teaching and learning because they define content without dictating style or consulting method and they can be achieved by using different skills and strategies (Box 1.1).

Chapter 6 describes our current formulation of the tasks of effective consulting: the thread that runs through the rest of the book.

Box 1.1 **The original consultation tasks (1984)**

1. To define the reasons for the patient's attendance, including:
   the nature and history of the problems
   their aetiology
   the patients' ideas, concerns and expectations
   the effects of the problems.
2. To consider other problems:
   continuing problems
   at risk factors.
3. With the patient, to choose an appropriate action for each problem.
4. To achieve a shared understanding of the problem with the patient.
5. To involve the patient in the management and to encourage him to accept appropriate responsibility.
6. To use time and resources appropriately:
   in the consultation
   in the long term.
7. To establish or maintain a relationship with the patient which helps to achieve the other tasks.

An approach to learning and teaching

In the original book we described an approach to learning and teaching that included:

◆ a clear, evidence based model of what was to be learned, the tasks for effective consultations
◆ a theoretical framework for effective teaching
◆ opportunities to practise and methods of observation, particularly video-recording
◆ methods for analysis and evaluation of a consultation (the map and rating scale)
◆ a method of giving effective feedback

This approach was based on a number of principles. The principles include

1. Everyone can improve their consultation skills.
2. Nearly all doctors have a range of sophisticated communication skills; though these are sometimes not used in the consultation.

3. People need to base new learning on their current understanding, so learners' understanding needs to be sought before teaching occurs.

4. Learning experiences should match the messages in the teaching, so patient-centred consulting is best taught using a learner-centred approach.

5. Different people learn in different ways so the teaching needs to have different methods, levels of abstraction and sources but the message needs to be consistent.

6. There are three steps towards effective skill development, namely: a clear understanding of what is to be learned, an opportunity to practise with feedback on performance, and opportunities to put the lessons into routine performance.

7. People develop more effectively when they have a clear idea of their strengths, a clear idea of what they need to improve and how that change can be achieved.

Subsequent experience in healthcare and in the industrial world, and our work with Donald McIntyre (Havelock *et al.* 1995) have served to confirm that these principles are robust and are suitable to wider application.

In the early 1980s, the use of video recording of real consultations for teaching purposes was new. As the technique has grown in popularity, the equipment has also improved beyond all recognition, making the logistics of producing useful video-recordings of consultations much simpler. It is now an acceptable technique to most doctors in primary care and is getting wider recognition in other medical disciplines. Since then, patient-centred consulting and learner-centred teaching have been developed and enhanced by many doctors, authors, researchers and teachers. In subsequent sections we discuss many outstanding contributions. We also describe how our own thinking has changed.

Since 1980, over 1000 doctors have been through our three-day course for learning and teaching on the consultation of which over 150 courses have been run throughout the United Kingdom and elsewhere. We have evaluated these courses and developed the teaching further. There has also been some criticism of some elements of our approach to teaching, such as the rules for feedback, often described as 'The Pendleton Rules'. This criticism has maintained that they confine the teaching and do not allow effective learning (Kurtz *et al.* 1998).

In Chapters 7–9 you will find our current approach to learning and teaching, including revisiting the rules for effective feedback. They are intended to be a practical guide for those who want to be involved in raising their own game and that of their colleagues.

In Chapters 10 and 11 you will find our concluding thoughts on dissemination and wider issues. We believe that the effect of 20 years of research and teaching is frustratingly small, and that there are still considerable challenges to be overcome if patient-centred medical care is to become the norm.

Nevertheless our passionate belief is that this is a goal that continues to be worthwhile and that the effort required of us all is easily justified.

Conclusion

This second book has been a long time coming! We have wanted to wait until we had something new to add to the debate. We also want to celebrate and recognize the outstanding contributions made in the field of effective consultation by so many authors from around the world. To borrow a quotation from Isaac Newton: 'If we see further, it is because we stand on the shoulders of giants'.

2 The cycle of care

'The consultation is the central act of medicine and as such it deserves to be understood' (Spence 1960). In the United Kingdom alone, it has been estimated that there may be as many as a million consultations per day. If the same ratios applied, then there would be roughly 4.5 million per day in the United States, 60,000 in New Zealand, half a million in Canada, and 2 million in Japan. Whatever the precise figures, medical consultations are common occurrences and most people in the industrialized countries will have between two and four consultations per year.

Medical care is a part of life and each consultation has a context. The sequence of events leading up to a consultation influence its content. The consultation, in its turn, has an impact and influences subsequent events for both doctor and patient. In the first book, we suggested a model to describe these antecedents and consequences for patients, the cycle of care (Pendleton 1983), which we used to derive our consultation tasks. We argued that a successful consultation was defined more by its effects than its processes. An effective consultation took account of those factors that resulted in the consultation, such as the clinical history of the problem and the patient's interpretations of events. An effective consultation also resulted in beneficial outcomes, such as reduction in the patient's concerns, adherence to the action plan developed in the consultation, and improvements in the patient's health. Not all good consultations can achieve ideal outcomes but those consultation processes that *regularly* succeed are effective.

The state of our understanding in 1984 allowed us to comment only on the patient's side of the cycle with any confidence. This chapter, which is the organizing framework for the first half of this book, outlines the model as we have now come to understand it. It is informed by a great deal of new thinking, described in later chapters, and it also comments on features that might become the subject of future study. The doctor's side is a little more explicit here than before and this accurately reflects a shift in our focus over the last 20 years.

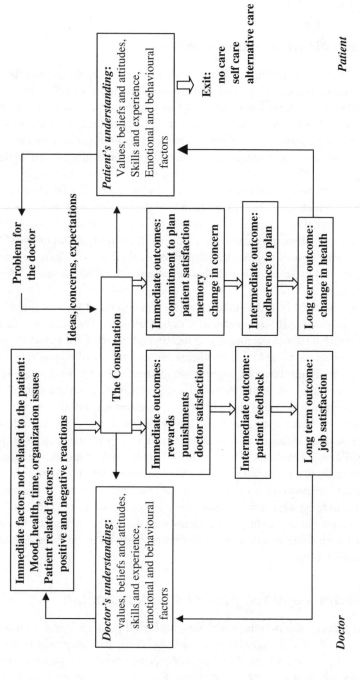

Fig. 2.1 The cycle of care.

The cycle as we now understand it

See Fig 2.1.

Antecedents of the consultation

Chapter 4 covers the patient's side of the cycle in some detail and describes its physical, psychological, and social dimensions. The patient's world is relatively well understood and has been researched in considerable detail. The doctor's side of the cycle has been rather less well researched and may be considered to be less well understood. Nevertheless, Chapter 5 draws together a mix of both empirical and theoretical pieces to elaborate our understanding of the doctor's world.

Antecedents on the patient's side of the cycle tend to be focused on *the problem* for which they are seeking help, and the reasons why they choose to seek help at that time. These reasons include their understanding of the possible nature of the problem, it's meaning to them, and their expectations of what help the doctor may be able to provide, often based on their previous experiences of health care. All these factors will also be influenced by the patient's cultural background.

Doctor's are likely to be influenced by some general factors including *cultural, professional, and personal issues*. Cultural influences include the expectations held about doctors in our society and the roles we expect them to fulfil. Professional issues include ethical and other rules of conduct, and the current state of beliefs about appropriate medical care. Chapter 3 considers these matters in more detail. Personal issues will vary from the state of the medical practice (the organization itself) and relationships within it, to the state of the doctor's home and family, and his or her personal health. In addition, there are personal issues that are bound up much more with the doctor's current workload and perceptions. These will include his or her mood, the current pressures of time, and the state in which the last patient left the room.

Other antecedents on the doctor's side are specifically related to the patient who is about to be seen. Since doctors are also human, we can expect that they will anticipate the arrival of some patients with delight and others with dread, and most with some reaction in between. The doctor's cycle is described in more detail in Chapter 5.

The doctor's and the patient's understanding

For many years, the popular view has contrasted patients' beliefs with the doctor's medical knowledge. David Tuckett and colleagues suggested an alternative (Tuckett *et al.* 1985). Their book described medical consultations as 'Meetings Between Experts' in which the doctor and the patient each brought specialist knowledge. The doctor could justly claim to know a great deal about how the body works, how diseases present and progress, how they should be investigated and how treated. The patient knows a great deal about him/herself: about the experience of the problem, about the personal values and needs which will govern how a problem is approached, about his/her lifestyle and the social context into which any proposed management plan has to fit. Both perspectives will influence the effectiveness with which any problem is addressed, and both perspectives need to find a place in the consultation.

For us, a consultation is a meeting between *people* in which each is usually trying to influence the other in some way. Each has specialist knowledge as the Tuckett team argued. Yet, each also has ideas and beliefs, feelings and motives, values and needs that they bring to the consultation. Thus, for us, the key concept for both doctor and patient is *Understanding*: the result of formal and informal learning, general and professional socialization, and the individual's upbringing and experience. It is a mix of cognition and affect: the thoughts and feelings that govern the doctor's and the patient's orientation to a consultation and help shape its contents.

Consequences of the consultation

There are very different types of outcomes that occur once a consultation has ended. For the patient, *immediate* outcomes include such factors as commitment to the management plan agreed in the consultation, his or her satisfaction with the consultation itself, his or her memory for what was said, and any change in the initial level of concern. One of the most widely researched *intermediate* patient outcomes is adherence to the proposed treatment (or management plan). We shall come to see in Chapter 4 that both consultation processes and some immediate outcomes affect patient adherence. Later, there is the *longer-term* outcome of change in the patient's health, which is to some extent governed by adherence to the proposed treatment. Finally, patients learn from their reflections on these experiences and so sustain or modify their *understanding*.

For the doctor, *immediate* outcomes include the pleasant and unpleasant consequences of certain aspects of their consultations. These form rewards and punishments that encourage or discourage certain consulting styles. When a practitioner zealously brings new approaches to an established practice, the patients' reactions to these differences may determine whether the doctor presses on with greater enthusiasm or drops the novel practices completely. Other immediate outcomes will include the doctor's satisfaction with the consultation and any immediate feedback the patient gives.

Longer-term outcomes for the doctor include the level of job satisfaction experienced. This is a prime determinant of motivation and morale, and can directly affect decision-making. Values are also relevant here and may change over time. Our approach to teaching, described in later chapters, reflects our concern with these broader issues. We also believe there is a great deal of research to be done on the relationship between immediate rewards and punishments, consultation satisfaction, longer-term job satisfaction, and the impact on the doctor's values and behaviour.

Summary

1. Consultations take place in a broader social and professional context which also fashions the dominant system of healthcare.

2. There are antecedents and consequences of all consultations for doctor and patient that influence the consultation's content and effectiveness.

3. Outcomes from consultations for doctor and patient can be placed in a sequence in which shorter-term outcomes influence later outcomes.

4. Doctors and patients make sense of their experiences of health and health care by developing their understanding. This forms the primary link between consultations.

3   The context of the consultation

Introduction

Doctors and patients and the nature of the consultations between them are profoundly influenced by the social and cultural context in which they take place. As practitioners and as teachers we need to be aware of these influences, and the ways that they may be changing over time. They have also influenced the model of the consultation and the cycle of care that is described in this book.

Beliefs about the causes of disease

Over the last century, the prevailing *medical model* has been that patients developed diseases which had defined causes and required diagnosis and treatment, preferably directed at the cause. This model has been extremely powerful. One example of this reductionist approach was Koch's postulates demonstrating the fact that the tubercle bacillus was the cause of a defined disease, tuberculosis, which had previously been described as an illness of phythis or consumption. This led to the development of specific treatments, including antibiotics.

Evidence for a *social model* was described by McKeown (1979), who pointed out that the remarkable decline in mortality from tuberculosis in the United Kingdom took place well before the development of these treatments and immunization. Instead it could be largely attributed to improvements in social conditions, which increased people's resistance to infection, and reduced their exposure to over crowded and unsanitary conditions. Medicine has also revised its view of the nature of susceptibility and resistance to disease. Good nutrition and hygiene remain important for developing resistance to infectious disease, particularly in children, but there is growing evidence that these factors in the early years can influence an individual's susceptibility to heart disease in later life (Barker *et al.* 2001).

The causes of disease can be understood most fully by considering *the whole person* in the context of their environment. For example, the conventional risk factors for heart disease, smoking, diet and lack of exercise are all dimensions of individual lifestyle. In addition there is growing evidence that social stresses, for example unemployment or employment in jobs over which the individual has little control, also increase that person's susceptibility to disease, particularly heart disease (Marmot *et al.* 1997).

The hope has been expressed that with our growing knowledge of human genetics we will soon be able to understand the relationships between the genome and our genetic predisposition to disease and the environmental factors that lead to it's expression. The phrase 'genetic engineering' implies that, with sufficient knowledge, this is a problem, which could be fixed. However the problems that face us in the practice of medicine will continue to be the relationship between the individual's lifestyle and their social situation and the effects that social inequalities have on health.

These problems affect the consultation in a number of ways. As we will describe in Chapter 4, understanding the patient includes not just the disease and it's pathological cause, but also the patient's lifestyle and the social factors that mould it. Second, it is important for medicine not to be sucked into 'victim blaming' where the patient is blamed for adopting unhealthy lifestyles, and is given advice which they do not have the capacity or resources to enact, and are then blamed again for failing to do so. The medical profession is unanimous in believing that cigarette advertising by large multinational companies encourages young people to take up a highly addictive habit. We also tend to get exasperated when our older patients fail to give up such a self-evidently unhealthy habit and blame them for it. We therefore need to be able to tailor our advice to that individual's needs and capacities.

The account given so far on the causes of disease remains scientific and reductionist, albeit with a wider view of the epidemiological factors involved. However, as society becomes more multicultural we need to recognize that many of our patients will have very different explanatory models for disease, ideas about illness and healing, and expectations of their doctors. This will also have, or should have, implications for the ways we train doctors to consult and assess their consultations.

Society's views on the nature of illness

Illness is a wider concept than disease and is defined in terms of the patient rather than an impersonal part of the body. It includes how the patient responds to the problem, how it affects their behaviour and relationships, and the meaning that they give to their experience.

Society's views of illness can define the roles to be expected of both patients and doctors in the consultation. Parsons' (1951) classic description of the *sick role* involved the expectations that patients should want to get well as quickly as possible and therefore to seek professional advice and cooperate with the doctor. In return they were allowed to shed some normal activities and responsibilities and be regarded as being in need of care. In Parsons' model, doctors are expected to apply a high degree of skill and knowledge to the problems of the illness, to act to promote the welfare of the patient and to be objective and emotionally detached. Doctors act as the gatekeeper to the sick role and this is sometimes formalized by the issue of medical certificates. This does not cause problems if the patient is seen to be fulfilling their part of the implied contract. However if the patient is not taking steps to get well as quickly as possible or adhering to medical advice, then the doctor can be cast in an authoritarian and judgemental role.

One important part of Parsons' definition of the role of the doctor is the provision of care, and by implication, not just the provision of cure. The growth of medical technology has enhanced the power of the medical profession at the risk of altering the nature of the relationship between the doctor and patient. One indicator of this is the growing trend to confine length of stay in hospital to only the time required to perform a technical procedure. It is in this environment medical students and junior doctors receive the large majority of their training. McWhinney (1995) has argued eloquently for a new paradigm of medical practice in which the duty to understand the patient's illness experience, and to relieve suffering, remains central to medical care.

Health and health care

During the last 50 years there has been a profound reassessment of both the meaning of health and the role of health services in 'producing' health. In 1948, the World Health Organization defined health as 'a complete state of physical, mental and social well being' and not merely the absence of disease and infirmity. In 1984, they expanded this to describe health as 'the extent to which an individual is able on the one hand to realize aspirations and satisfy needs: and on the other hand to change or cope with the environment'. Health is therefore seen as a resource for everyday life and not the object of living: it is a positive concept emphasizing social and personal resources as well as physical capacities. These conditions may seem utopian and reflecting the decline in infectious diseases and the growing prevalence of long-term chronic illness. However this view of health as a resource, maximizing freedom of choice and the opportunities for gaining satisfaction from living, is one that is widely shared. Labonte (1993), as part of the Toronto Declaration, identified six components of good health. These were:

◆ feeling vital and full of energy.

◆ having good social relationships

◆ experiencing a sense of control over one's life and living conditions

◆ being able to do things one enjoys

◆ having a sense of purpose in life

◆ experiencing being part of a community

Individuals have a range of views of what health means to them. Crawford (1984) explored this and described two broad categories of belief. The first he described as *health as control*, leading a healthy lifestyle, having regular medical check-ups and not having any diseases, which he equated with the self-improving thread in American culture. The other description was as *health as release* 'being able to do what I want to do when I want to do it without worrying' which he equated with the culture of consuming the good life. Doctors need to recognize where their own beliefs sit on this continuum and how that influences their views of their patients. Do we really believe that patients who consult us frequently are healthy? We also need to establish the views of our individual patients, particularly in relation to lifestyle.

Illich (1976) has criticized the medical profession for using this broader account of health to extend its interventions into more and more areas of normal life creating medical dependence or iatrogenesis. However, an alternative view is that if health can be defined as a capacity required to make choices, and to be in control of one's life, then one of the roles of health care is to help people expand and develop those capacities. This means that the provision of information, the discussion of options, and the promotion of choice and autonomy become central to our tasks in each of our consultations.

Within these broad aims there remains the need to offer patients those elements of medical care that may improve their health. In our 'First World' society it is easy to lose sight of the importance of a health care system that enables all children, irrespective of their income, to be offered appropriate immunizations, that screens women for cancer, and detects high blood pressure and other risk factors for heart disease in the whole population. This can be achieved by systematic invitations to the registered population, but it is well known that those in greatest need are least likely to accept. However, these same people are more likely to consult their doctor. This means that every consultation is an opportunity to detect risk factors and to offer opportunistic care (Stott and Davis 1979).

The structure of health care systems

Probably the most profound influence of society on the consultation is the structure of the health care system itself. This book has been written from the perspective of primary care, though the approach to the consultation and it's teaching is, in our experience, applicable to the whole of health care.

Primary care is the *first point of contact* with the health care system for patients with problems, and the symptoms and illnesses they present are relatively disorganized. This is the first attempt by a professional to make sense of them and that this is usually done without recourse to much medical technology. The large majority of symptoms that patients experience are not presented to doctors at all and the large of majority of illness episodes presented to primary care are managed within primary care. Primary care therefore has a crucial role of helping patients understand their symptoms and enhancing their ability to manage problems themselves.

In a system where the relationship between primary care and secondary care is one of *referral*, the nature of the problems presented and the expectations of doctors are very different. Marshall Marinker's aphorism is that 'secondary care reduces uncertainty, explores possibility and marginalises error whilst Primary care tolerates uncertainty, explores probability and marginalises danger' (Marinker 1996). The gatekeeper role has traditionally been seen as a way of ensuring that patients receive appropriate specialist advice and investigation, but also protects them from over-investigation, over-treatment, and over-medicalization of illness.

The *gatekeeper role*, however, has assumed additional significance as health care systems attempt to contain escalating health care costs. Whilst this may have been implicit for many years, it has now become very explicit. With development of managed care and cash limited budgets there can be a conflict of interest between the doctor's duty to provide, and to obtain, all necessary care for the individual patient, and act as the patient's advocate within the health care system; and the doctor's responsibility to use health care resources to the best advantage of the whole population. Wherever possible it is desirable that this negotiation takes place openly and explicitly both with individual patients and groups representing patients' interests.

Probably the most precious resource that doctors ration is that of their own *time*. We are totally accustomed to the idea that we set limits on the length of our booking times for consultations, even though this varies greatly between different countries and health care systems. However, with the growing evidence of increased effectiveness with longer consultations (Freeman *et al.* 2002), having adequate time, and using it to best effect, becomes a major determinant of the quality of care in the consultation.

Within a prepaid health care system such as the British National Health Service, doctors are responsible for providing care for a defined list of patients, and negotiations about time and workload take place with the employing or contracting authority. The issue ultimately comes down to the size of the population served by each doctor. In a fee for service system, the patient in theory has a greater degree of control but there is clearly an incentive for the doctor to see as many patients as he or she can. This dichotomy can also be seen in the extent to which in a socialized or prepaid system, the patients are seen to be receiving a charitable good whilst in a fee for service system the patients are seen as customers. On the other hand, a prepaid system can liberate doctors from the need to obtain fees for repeat attendances from each patient and can therefore provide more disinterested advice and encourage more independence on the patient's part.

Another key element of the health care system that affects the consultation is the degree to which it promotes *continuity of care (care by the same doctor on subsequent occasions)*. The cycle of care, described in Chapter 2, essentially describes the patient's experience of repeated encounters with health care. Hjortdahl (Hjortdahl and Laerum 1992) demonstrated the benefits of these encounters being with the same physician and Pereira-Gray (1998) has described how, in British general practice, patients on an average have over three quarters of an hour of contact with their doctor each year. This is an opportunity for the doctor and patient to get to know each other and develop a growing relationship. Balint (1957) described the potential for this relationship to be 'a mutual investment company which can yield dividends as the relationship deepens'. However, it remains possible for a succession of doctors to provide consistent care. Each consultation is an opportunity to develop patients' health understanding and their expectations of consultations.

An increasingly important part of both formal and informal health care systems is the development of *alternative sources of information* for patients other than face-to-face contact with their doctor. Some of these are well established, for example patient information leaflets and leaflets included with medication. There is an increasing concern about the quality of much of this information, particularly its readability and the extent to which it is evidence based (Coulter *et al.* 1999). Giving patients such information, particularly in the form of decision aids that encourage patient choice, can encourage patients to read and reflect before coming to important decisions (O'Connor *et al.* 1999).

Health information is now widely available to those who have access to libraries and the Internet. Doctors may perceive it as a challenge to their authority and to their role as the sole source of their patients' information, but on the whole this is a positive development. However, it can widen the gap in society between those who are well educated and informed and those that are not. Paradoxically, doctors are much more willing to enter into a dialogue with patients who are already well informed and ask relevant questions, which can exacerbate this problem still further. Helping patients obtain, understand, and evaluate information is going to become a very important part of the doctor's role in the future.

Professional regulation

Society impinges explicitly on the doctor–patient relationship through its mechanisms for professional regulation. The General Medical Council in the United Kingdom has included aspects of communication in its statement of Good Medical Practice (General Medical Council 1998), including listening to patients, informing them in ways that can be understood, and involving patients in decisions about their care. The General Medical Council also recommended in 'Tomorrow's Doctors' (General Medical Council 1993), that communication skills teaching should be included throughout the medical curriculum. Most medical students now receive such training, and an increasing number are examined on their ability to be able to communicate as part of the certified examinations.

Increasingly, doctors will be held to account for their adherence to such standards by mechanisms of professional self-regulation and revalidation. In the United Kingdom these mechanisms are only effectively in place for teachers of general practice who may have video recordings of their consultations reviewed as part of their assessment for re-approval as trainers. However, if re-validation of all doctors is based on some form of regular re-assessment of performance, and the consultation is central to our work as general practitioners, then methods of assessment of effectiveness in the consultation will have to be used. This will be an opportunity to define effectiveness as the extent to which tasks important to patients are achieved.

The ethical framework

The practice of medicine is also guided by an ethical framework, partly generated from within the profession, but increasingly externally reinforced. The dialogue on ethics in medicine has been strongly influenced by the work of Beauchamp and Childress (1979). They presented four principles: respect for autonomy, beneficence, non-maleficence and justice.

They defined *autonomy* as 'when people act intentionally with understanding and without controlling influences that determine their actions'. This definition introduces two important concepts, that of informed understanding and that of freedom of choice. One question is whether autonomy, so defined, is a natural right for all people, or whether it is a capacity that may or may not be present but which doctors have a duty to respect and develop.

If it is regarded as a natural right, then respect for autonomy must transcend the other ethical principles, which can lead to difficulties, which will be discussed later. If autonomy is regarded as a capacity which depends both on the possession of information and understanding and also on the freedom to be able to make, and to implement choices, then respecting a patient's autonomy involves developing their understanding and enabling their effectiveness. This is a central task for our consultations.

The principle of *beneficence* is that the primary obligation of doctors is to act for the benefit of their patients. This can be interpreted as meaning that the doctor should make decisions about management as patients, particularly when ill, wish their doctors to take responsibility for making decisions relating to their health. It can further be argued that the patient can never match the doctors' knowledge and training, and that it is important for the patient to have faith in their doctors as this is beneficial in the healing process. However, there is a growing body of evidence which indicates that patients who are informed about their health and involved in making choices, look after their health better and have improved health outcomes (Greenfield *et al.* 1985). Encouraging patients to be involved in choices about their own care can therefore be seen as a way of achieving beneficence, acting for the good of the patient.

The other difficulty with beneficence as a guiding principle is to distinguish it from paternalism. Paternalism can include the withholding of information from the patient and a failure to respect the patient's values, particularly about the desired outcomes of their care.

On first sight the principle of *non-maleficence*, or doing no harm, appears less problematic. However, difficulties arise when it is in conflict with other principles, for example doctors defending their right and responsibility to prescribe certain drugs on the grounds that only they fully understand the harm that they can do. Where do the boundaries lie when patients wish to choose to receive antibiotics for viral infections or long-term prescriptions for sleeping tablets?

Avoiding harm may also involve recognizing the iatrogenic effects of labelling people as diseased and increasing peoples' dependence on health care. There is a particular duty to avoid harm in the field of screening and preventive medicine. Healthy individuals are invited to submit themselves to tests that may lead to further investigations and added anxieties, sometimes only to be told later that they are in fact normal, or to be told that they need treatment which the profession presumes is for their benefit.

The final principal, *justice*, is concerned with fairness between people, which can relate both to medical practice and the use of health care resources, but also to peoples' wider life experience. The utilitarian principle of doing the greatest good for the greatest number may again be in conflict with the desire to do the very best for an individual.

Understanding these four principles and their implications can be helpful in two ways. First, our statements of purpose in the consultation, or tasks, needs to be informed by these ethical principles. Second, they can help us understand and resolve the dilemmas that face us in many of our consultations.

The legal framework

These ethical issues are sometimes enshrined in the law, which has been particularly concerned with the issue of *informed consent to treatment*. The law has attempted to help the medical profession balance its duties between absolute respect for the patient's autonomy and their desire to benefit and not to harm the patient.

These issues were considered very fully in the courts in the United Kingdom in the case of Amy Sidaway in which a patient underwent an operation on her cervical vertebrae to rid herself of recurrent pain and unfortunately sustained damage to the spinal cord leading to severe disability. Her case was not that the operation had been performed negligently, but that if she had been fully informed of the risks of the procedure, she would not have undertaken it. On the one hand it was argued that patients have a right to choose what should happen to their bodies and to do this they require information on all material risks. On the other hand it was argued that patients can never be as fully informed as the doctor, and that volunteering information about remote risks may unduly alarm the patient and put them off the treatment.

It was also argued that there was a responsible body of medical opinion that would not have disclosed remote risks. This view was criticized by Lord Scarman who gave a dissenting judgement on the grounds that 'the court should not allow medical opinion as what is best for the patient to override the patients' rights to decide for himself whether he will submit to the treatment offered to him'. The majority judgement, however, found in favour of Mrs Sidaway's surgeon and UK law remains that it is the medical profession's responsibility to decide what information is material for the patient to know (Sidaway *v.* Bethlem Royal Hospital 1985).

However, one of the issues raised by the 'Bristol case' (Smith 1998), in which two paediatric surgeons were found to have had unduly poor results from their paediatric cardiac surgery, was the way in which risk was explained to patients. Clearly, public and professional opinion has followed Lord Scarman in shifting away from respecting medical paternalism and towards expecting fully informed choice.

One aspect of informed choice that causes particular problems for doctors is when the results of a particular intervention are thought to benefit the community as well as the individual patient. Examples of this are childhood immunizations that create population or 'herd' immunity, screening procedures such as cervical cytology to reduce the burden of cancer or evidence based treatments such as anticoagulants for patients with atrial fibrillation to prevent strokes. What all these have in common is a belief that these treatments will benefit the individual but also an expectation that early treatment or prevention of disease will contain health care costs. Targets are set for population coverage, and these pressures can influence the doctor to manipulate the patient to obtain consent rather than promote informed choice. In our view, we need to move to a position in which informed choice is a key outcome measure for effective preventive care.

Summary

1. It is as difficult to understand the consultation without being aware of the social and cultural context in which it takes place, as it is to understand the patient without knowing about their life and work.

2. These influences have helped us to define the nature of the doctor–patient relationship and the tasks to be achieved in a consultation. The emphasis on understanding the whole patient and their illness experience and sharing information, decisions and responsibility with patients stems from our view of the role of medicine in a modern liberal society.

3. However, the fact that amongst our patients there will be a wide variety of culture and values as well as social and illness experience means that

exploring and respecting the individuals values and beliefs is an essential pre-cursor to decisions about management and care.

4. If we accept the principle of respecting the patient's autonomy and regard it as a capacity that can be developed, then the provision of information, the development of understanding and the enablement of choice can be seen as central to our role as doctors.

5. They should also become central in our teaching, in our assessment of professional performance, and in the legal and contractual framework within which we work.

4 Understanding the patient

In Chapter 2, we argued that there are inputs for each medical consultation that influence both its content and outcomes. For the patient, these inputs comprise physical, psychological, and social dimensions, and the interplay between them. The physical dimension includes the vicissitudes of everyday sensation: how the patient feels. The psychological dimension includes the complex web of ideas, beliefs, emotions, expectations, and coping mechanisms that permeate the patient's world and through which it is perceived and understood. The social dimension is even more disparate and ranges from religious and demographic influences at the most general to the more immediate and specific influences of family and friends.

This chapter will attempt to understand the patient by considering the contextual elements for each consultation. It will consider the inputs to, and outcomes of, medical consultations from the patient's perspective. This chapter along with Chapter 5, which considers the doctor's perspective, and Chapter 6, which focuses on consultation processes, covers the entire input-process-outcome model that comprises the cycle of care.

Inputs to the consultation

Physical issues

Everyday experience of health and illness is unspectacular. Our experience varies. One day we will wake up with a headache, the next we will not. Some days we seem to have more energy than others. Some nights we sleep better than others. There is a broad range of normal experiences that we do not particularly notice. Yet there are also experiences that we notice, worry about, and cause us to seek help.

Few physical experiences trigger the same behaviour in everyone. David Hannay (1979) studied the health experiences of an inner city population and demonstrated that most physical experiences can be labelled as symptoms or not, depending on the point of view of the individual to whom the experience happened.

The reasons for a consultation are not to be understood in an account of 'symptoms' alone. The reasons a person becomes a patient are to be found in his or her understanding of personal experiences, and in the effects triggered by both the symptoms and their interpretation. Diagnosis thus becomes a broader notion and management of the problem contains a greater variety of possibilities.

Psychological issues

Some illnesses such as anxiety and depression are labelled as predominantly psychological but have physical components. In others, psychological factors are able to cause physical ill-health directly and a lexicon of terms has been coined to express this experience. Conditions such as tension headaches or irritable bowel syndrome may be described as psychosomatic or psychogenic when their origin is essentially psychological. Other conditions, such as asthma, may be exacerbated by psychological factors, and in others the psychological reaction to physical disease is a major component of the patient's illness. *Somatisation* refers to the tendency for emotional pressures to manifest themselves as physical symptoms (Balint 1957; Grol 1989).

There are therefore powerful psychological factors at work in *all* experiences of illness, and in all consultations, as Michael Balint first pointed out in 1957. These include cognitive factors such as ideas and beliefs, emotional factors such as feelings and concerns, and behavioural factors such as coping mechanisms. They are all featured, moreover, in patients' accounts of their experiences or narratives.

Ideas and beliefs

At the time of writing our first book, the dominant models in the emerging field of health psychology were cognitive models. Attempts were made to explain help seeking behaviour, behaviour in the consultation, behaviour following medical consultations and preventative or health promoting behaviours in terms of cognitive models.

The Health Belief Model (HBM; Becker 1974) has five elements:

1. Health motivation: people vary in their overall interest in health and in their motivation to look after themselves.
2. Perceived vulnerability: the *perceived* likelihood of contracting any particular condition.
3. Perceived seriousness: if any condition were to be contracted, this element refers to the *perceived* seriousness of the consequences.
4. Perceived costs and benefits: the advantages and disadvantages of treating or not treating any specific condition.
5. Cues to action: the factors that trigger a set of beliefs or activities.

The HBM usefully demonstrated the subjectivity of these various factors and has been used successfully to predict help seeking, compliance with medical advice, and preventive health behaviour. A central issue highlighted by the HBM is 'congruence'. Patients are less likely to follow advice in a consultation that is incongruent with their health beliefs. They are also less likely to remember it (Becker and Maiman 1975).

These factors influence the consultation. The reasons the patient has consulted is determined in large part by his or her beliefs. The credibility of any diagnosis is influenced by the patient's beliefs. The likelihood of remembering or following through on advice given is influenced by the patient's beliefs. Thus, as George Bernard Shaw argued in 'The doctor's dilemma': the doctor who remains ignorant of the patient's beliefs is lost.

A similar cognitive model is Health Locus Of Control (Rotter 1966). The concept of Locus of Control refers to the specific beliefs an individual may hold about his or her potency in controlling significant events. An internal controller believes that his destiny is in his own hands. An external controller believes that external factors control her destiny, whether this is such a general matter as fate or other powerful people.

It is proposed that patients differ considerably in their belief in their own capacity to influence their health, and empirical validation of these ideas is strong. Fatalists tend not to look after themselves, whereas internal controllers do. Internal controllers are more likely to ask their doctor for information, take their medication appropriately, keep to a diet, and successfully give up smoking. They are also more likely to keep medical appointments (Wallston and Wallston 1978).

Feelings and concerns

When most patients visit most doctors, there is an element of concern that has given rise to the visit. Our own research demonstrated the pervasiveness of patient's concerns (Pendleton 1981) though even a casual observer of medical practice will not need further proof. More recently, Joe Kai (1996) has elucidated the matter of parental concerns about their children's health. He demonstrated the link of that concern with their sense of control over their children's health and their need to cope effectively with the threat of illness to their children.

Feelings are also outcomes from consultations. The conversation with the doctor may have had an effect on the patient's level of concern and/or the patient's commitment to the recommended course of action.

Ironically, though concerns are pervasive in the experience of most patients, it has been known for some time that they are seldom adequately explored in most medical consultations. A significant proportion of patients' concerns are not discussed in their consultations and the Royal College of General Practitioners in the United Kingdom has evidence from their membership examinations that patients' feelings are seldom explored in consultations (Tate *et al.* 1999). Yet it is the complex interplay of ideas and concerns that is most relevant for medical consultations. Indeed, they do not exist in isolation from each other, and they influence the behaviour of doctor and patient.

Self regulation: the integration of approaches

Whole person medicine is a cornerstone of primary care, and for good reason. Yet, however holistic the ideal, both practice and research are needed to analyse and work with its elements, though some more recent models have allowed us to grapple with more of the complexities of the whole person. Ideas and beliefs, feelings and concerns are organized into a coherent and self sustaining whole that both influence specific coping mechanisms and are influenced by them, (Leventhal and Cameron 1987). This is the Self Regulatory Model or SRM, and it is dynamic rather than static. Its elements are structured around five themes or questions in the patient's mind:

(1) identity: what is it?
(2) timeline: how long will it last?
(3) cause: what caused it?
(4) consequences: how will it/has it affected me?
(5) cure/control: can it be cured or controlled?

The self-regulatory model (Fig 4.1) proposes that internal stimuli (such as a physical sensation) and/or external stimuli (such as an article in a newspaper), may provoke cognitive, emotional and behavioural responses. The cognitive response is in the form of ideas and beliefs that constitute the patient's 'Representation of the problem'. This provokes coping mechanisms in the patient, which the model calls an 'Action plan for coping with the problem' and also some means of making a rough and ready evaluation of the adequacy of the plan, dubbed 'Appraisal' in the model.

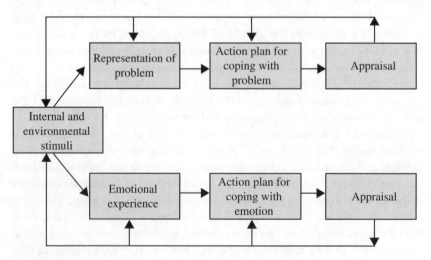

Fig. 4.1 The self-regulatory model (Leventhal and Cameron 1987).

There is a parallel emotional response. The 'Emotional experience' is the feelings and concerns provoked. An 'Action plan for coping with the emotion' is also set up that is appropriate to the intensity and effect of the feelings and it too is monitored for effectiveness in dealing with the emotional experience by some form of 'Appraisal'.

These form an integrated and self-sustaining response to an event or a problem. The specific ideas, concerns, and behavioural responses to the trigger determine the global approach to the problem taken by the patient and predict subsequent attempts to deal with the issue. When the cognitive and emotional responses are compatible, the patient will act more consistently and more predictably. When they are incompatible or even in conflict, the patient will act more unpredictably.

Thus, on being told that a troublesome cough is actually asthma, the athlete may become overwhelmed with anxiety and thoroughly depressed by the prospect. He has told himself that it lasts forever, and though he does not know what has caused it, he knows that it makes people weedy and breathless, and is incurable. The action plan for coping with the emotions (denial) may so overwhelm any action plan for treating the condition that he both fails to attend to the details of the treatment recommendations and to follow through with the inhaler therapy.

Narratives

Patients' open-ended narratives also convey the richness of their experiences, and a detailed methodology has arisen for the exploration of narrative both in the consultation and in research. One of the most succinct summaries of the narrative approach has been provided by Jeanne and David Smith (Personal communication 1999):

> The narrative approach regards patient accounts as interpretations of patient experiences. People live in realities they have constructed symbolically. These symbols embody the meanings that experiences have for us. We can discover those meanings by examining the stories. Meanings are revealed in a number of ways:
>
> ♦ By what is selected by the story teller as important enough to relate as opposed to what is not thought to be important enough to tell about.
> ♦ By the way the descriptions of various characters reveal what is important and unimportant, good and bad, desirable and undesirable, etc.
> ♦ By the way the plot of the story is unfolded demonstrating what events have most importance and what values are assigned to various actions, events and outcomes.
> ♦ By the emotion displayed in the para-language [non-verbal communication] used by the story teller to reveal the intensity of meaning during the narration.

- By the emotion revealed in the figures of speech, especially metaphors used to emphasise and characterise the elements of the story.

This emphasis on narrative has been expanded in a series of articles and books (Greenhalgh and Hurwitz 1998) to include teaching and other approaches to patients' narrative. There is a database collected of patient experiences to aid greater understanding by both patients of their conditions and to increase the insight of doctors (Hexheimer *et al.* 2000).

William Osler's dictum to listen to the patient because he's trying to tell you the diagnosis could be expanded into advice to listen for all the richness of the patient's experience in the patient's story. Patients tell compelling stories to communicate their perceptions and swap stories to construct their sense of reality. Doctors relate statistics but without the persuasive force of the stories the patients relate. Doctors would do well to learn to relate counter stories in their consultations to combat the tales told by the patients: to set up a dissonant voice that compels re-evaluation.

Patients' expectations

We have seen how the HBM and the SRM explain the origin of expectations. In the case of the HBM, expectations are part of the analysis of costs and benefits of treating or not treating the condition. In the case of the SRM, expectations are part of the action plan and they are modified in the light of experience of (appraisal of) the action plan(s) implemented.

Expectations can be seen in day-to-day practice also. Patients form expectations about the condition, about the consultation, and about how it should be treated. Consider the following example:

> A man of 42 experiences pains in his chest while playing golf. These pains are relatively minor and are dismissed as unimportant. The pains recur while he is working in the garden. He takes a short rest to see if they will go away. The pain stops. After several days, back on the golf course, the pain reappears, and he considers the possibility that something may be wrong with him. He knows that he has been working hard lately and that he has been feeling rather weak, and the thought occurs that he may be falling ill. Chest pains are seldom good news. He mentions them to his wife who encourages him to see the doctor. He knows that chest pains may signify something seriously wrong and he is concerned that the doctor may overly restrict his normally active life. Nevertheless, he knows that he should see the doctor and he makes an appointment. After all, his father used to complain of pains in the chest, and he died of carcinoma of the oesophagus.

This man has thought about his health to a considerable extent. He has first ignored the problem, then done nothing about it, and then talked it over with his wife. He has two possible representations of the problem: either the pains are caused by muscle strain which will be short lived, caused by exertion, which will do little more than irritate and restrict him but that will be self-limiting. Or it may be oesophageal cancer, which will be terminal and which is incurable. His ideas and concerns are clear. He expects the doctor to consider these possibilities and examine him accordingly, after all, the same doctor cared for his father some 15 years ago and was with him when he died.

Patients' expectations derive from their representation of the problem and their experience of medical care. Their expectations of medical care govern their approach to such matters as whether or not they want to be involved in making choices about their care or want to be passive in the process (Coulter 1997; McKinstry 2000), about whether or not they want to receive a prescription and about the specific actions they want their doctor to take in considering their problem, investigating it and making a diagnosis. Perhaps even more significantly, Nicky Britten (Britten and Ukoumunne 1997) has shown that doctors are also strongly influenced by their perceptions of the patient's expectations—in this case in relation to the patient's perceived expectations for a prescription.

Thus, patients approach their consultations with an understanding of their problems, feelings about it, and expectations about the condition and how it needs to be addressed. Such an approach may be incomplete, rudimentary, and inaccurate or it may be coherent, well informed and entirely consistent with current medical opinion. Yet the patient's representation of the problem, his or her feelings and concerns about it, and the associated action plans for dealing with it are currently governing his or her behaviour. Any consultation that does not explore these matters is likely to be ineffective.

Social issues

Health and illness are labels we apply to a broad range of experiences. They are not objectively defined but subjectively. Disease is a more objective issue but even disease may be influenced by social and psychological factors. Demography (usually poverty) is a powerful determinant of the probability that an individual will or will not contract a disease, and of life expectancy even in an industrialized country (Black 1980). Religious beliefs can also influence susceptibility to physical threat. Curses can make people ill and miracles can cure representing the triumph of faith over adversity.

Insights about social issues derive from the study of populations. Two significant social influences on consultations are *values* and *norms*. Values are relatively abstract shared beliefs. Norms are more concrete ways of thinking; feeling and acting that derive from values. Both values and norms are learned from, and sustained by, membership of a social group. The social group in question may be as large as 'the industrialized nations' or as small as 'my family' but the influence is noticeable and needs to be understood.

Since doctors and patients usually come from different social groups, neither can easily use their own experiences to predict the other's. Doctors working in poor areas may find that their own time horizons differ hugely from those of their patients. The doctor may plan his or her financial security by taking the long-term view of investments and may take on a 25 year mortgage without a second thought. The patient may live a much more hand-to-mouth existence and have trouble thinking much further ahead than the next week's wages. In this case, what are the chances that the patient will take a similar view of advice to quit smoking in pregnancy—advice that appears eminently sensible to the doctor?

Doctors also acquire values and norms from their training, whether through conscious instruction, role modelling, or the gradual implementation of social reinforcement for conformity to the group's expectations. In these ways, doctors learn how to play the role of 'doctor' (see Chapter 5). There is also a 'patient' role, which has its own different rules. These roles, acquired and stabilized over time, become mutually sustaining. Indeed, Boreham and Gibson (1978) demonstrated that both doctors and patients generally agreed about what was appropriate behaviour for each party to play in their role, and that this agreement was around an active doctor and a reactive patient. If consultations are more effective when patients are more active, as we shall argue below, then it will be necessary to overcome a large measure of social learning.

Social factors also influence the decision to seek a doctor's help. David Tuckett (1976) reviews the evidence that:

> Individuals have symptoms much of the time, and that dealing with them, particularly by self-medication, is a day-to-day activity ... individuals visit the doctor on average for only one out of about ten symptoms they suffer ... when they do go, these symptoms have not necessarily got worse ... their motives for going and what they want from the doctor may often have more to do with some change in their social circumstances than with any change in symptoms

Social factors similarly affect the outcomes of consultations. Any management plan agreed in the consultation has to be applied by the individual in his social setting. In addition, the way doctors and patients judge whether a particular outcome is successful is dependent on their values and norms. David Tuckett (1976) illustrates the matter with reference to a range of possible outcomes after amputation of a patient's leg, thus:

(1) the operation scar has healed well and the patient can leave hospital;

(2) the cancer seems to be spreading to the rest of the body;

(3) he uses a wheelchair in preference to his artificial leg;

(4) he has lost his former job and is now unemployed; and

(5) his wife, disappointed at being married to a 'cripple' has left him.

Since insights about these social factors derive from studies of populations, in much the same way as does epidemiological research, it is crucial to recognize that simple generalizations are dangerous. Probabilities may suggest useful hypotheses but individuals differ and hypotheses are to be tested. The doctor's task is to understand and use these factors in the management of the consultation and the patient.

Outcomes from the consultation

The cycle of care (Chapter 2) demonstrates the variety of different outcomes from consultations. There are:

- immediate outcomes such as patient satisfaction
- intermediate outcomes such as patient compliance or adherence to the management plan
- longer-term outcomes such as changes in the patient's health, and
- the growth of the patient's understanding of his or her health and in the ability to look after it.

These were covered in the outline in our first book (Pendleton *et al.* 1984). By contrast Beckman *et al.* (1989) added a further category, *process outcomes*, by which they meant the effects of styles of communication on the consultation itself—strictly an output rather than an outcome as we shall see in Chapter 6.

At the time of writing the first book the evidence was already clear that outcomes of various kinds affect one another. It was clear, for example, that patient satisfaction and memory of the doctor's communication affected compliance. Fitzpatrick *et al.* (1983), in a longitudinal study of patients attending neurology out-patients for non-organic headache, found that the main factor related to reduction in symptoms was the patients' satisfaction with the consultation, and in particular being given information and advice that related to their concerns. This enabled them to make sense of their symptoms and achieve a sense of control over their illness.

Since then, the determinants of compliance, both in the consultation and elsewhere, have become better understood. The evidence will be reviewed briefly here, and some will be covered in greater depth below in Chapter 6. There has also been a development of the long-standing debate about the appropriateness of the term 'compliance'. It is covered briefly in the section on intermediate outcomes later in this chapter.

Immediate outcomes

By immediate outcomes we mean those effects of a consultation that may be discussed and researched at the end of the consultation. Here we shall cover the immediate outcomes of patient satisfaction, changes in patient concern, patient memory and understanding of the messages and recommendations received, and their commitment to the management plan.

Satisfaction

There is a wealth of evidence on the correlates of patient satisfaction. Of particular relevance here, Hall and colleagues (1988) analysed 41 such studies and found that there were significant positive correlations between patient satisfaction and three aspects of physician behaviour:

1. Giving information, particularly about the problem, its significance, and its treatment.

2. Partnership building, for example encouraging the patient to talk and asking for the patient's ideas and opinions.

3. 'Positive talk', expressing agreement, giving encouragement or reassurance, and showing understanding and concern.

Social conversation about non-medical matters had little effect, and there was a negative correlation with the proportion of question asked by the physicians.

Williams *et al.* (1995) similarly reviewed over 40 studies of patient satisfaction and showed more equivocal findings. Certainly information provision by the doctor was positively associated with patient satisfaction, as was patient information giving, though high levels of closed questions seemed to produce more negative results. Unsurprisingly, doctors' friendliness, courtesy, and expression of warm and positive feelings in consultations were positively associated with patient satisfaction, whereas the expression of negative feelings (irritation, anger, etc.) were associated with dissatisfaction.

More recently, Kinnersley *et al.* (1999) demonstrated that patient-centred styles of consulting are associated with increased patient satisfaction. Patient satisfaction has also been associated with increased patient compliance, as we shall see below, but Winefield and colleagues (1995) showed that there was little correlation between patient satisfaction and doctor satisfaction with specific consultations.

There is increasing interest in other outcomes such as patient enablement (Howie *et al.* 1997) and shared medical decision-making (Elwyn, Edwards, and Kinnersley 1999). There is also an increasing focus on more direct changes in patient health status such as the level of control of diabetes and hypertension, and quality adjusted life years as a means of comparing outcome benefits of different medical procedures.

Concern

Many concerns are not communicated in medical consultations and yet there is clear evidence that satisfaction, concerns and health outcomes are related. In a primary care study of 716 consultations involving a sore throat, Little and colleagues (2001) demonstrated that patients who were more satisfied got better more quickly, and satisfaction related strongly to how well the doctor dealt with the patient's concerns.

In an earlier study of primary care consultations in the United Kingdom, it was found that neither the level of the patient's concern, nor any changes in that level, were related to the patient's memory for the communicated knowledge or advice in the consultation (Pendleton 1981).

Memory and understanding

The matter of patients' memory for medical advice is controversial and some-what confusing. Philip Ley (1979), asserted that patients forget around 50 per cent of what they are told, but neither Tuckett and colleagues (1985) nor Pendleton (1981) were able to replicate the findings. Indeed, both authors claim that patients remember the vast majority of the 'important' information they are told. Ley (1988) repeated the 50 per cent memory loss claim, and also asserted that medical information was not well understood. This claim is less controver-sial, and, on balance, it seems safe to conclude that it is important to attempt to check patients' understanding of the information they are told.

Commitment to the management plan

In view of the particular prominence of compliance/adherence as a subject for study, it is surprising that there have been few studies of building commitment to the agreed management plans. The evidence for patient involvement in decision-making will be reviewed in the following section, but involvement and commit-ment are correlated. One welcome and relevant addition to the literature has been the investigation of so-called motivational consulting (Miller 1983) based on Albert Bandura's self efficacy theory of behaviour change (Bandura 1977).

Enablement

John Howie and colleagues have more recently proposed a helpful new measure of a consultation's immediate outcomes. Their view is that patients need to leave a consultation feeling enabled by it, and recommend a measure of enable-ment as an indicator of quality of care. Their research has demonstrated the potential of a patient enablement index (PEI) as a quality measure that is related to, but different from, general patient satisfaction (Howie *et al.* 1998).

Compliance/adherence: the principal intermediate outcome

One outcome of the process of decision making in the consultation is whether the patient adheres to the advice or takes the treatment afterwards. This has tra-ditionally been described as compliance, but the term has been criticized as a concept on the grounds that it implies control by the doctor rather than patient choice. Generally, the term 'adherence' is preferred to compliance because this can describe adherence to a shared and agreed decision or plan. The Royal Pharmaceutical Society (1996) has recommended the term 'concordance' and in our view this nicely describes the achievement of a shared decision or 'concordat'. Yet concordance cannot substitute for the term adherence or compliance with that decision. We therefore use the term 'adherence to an agreed plan' and include both issues of compliance with medication and with advice about behavioural change.

As Stimpson and Webb (1975) pointed out:

> The crucial paradox . . . is that in the consultation the doctor makes the treatment decisions; after the consultation, decision making lies with the patient.

These matters have formed the basis of a great deal of research, much of which was conducted in the 1970s and 1980s. Most of the original research was of poor quality but more recent studies have been excellent, showing both how and why non-adherence happens, and how adherence can be improved somewhat.

For now, it is worthy of our attention that adherence to advice about medical treatment is relatively poor, irrespective of the condition and its seriousness. When it comes to lifestyle advice, compliance often falls to single percentage figures (Butler *et al.* 1996). Additionally, in a systematic review of randomized trials aimed at improving adherence to treatment, Haynes *et al.* (1996) concluded that even the most effective interventions did not lead to substantial improvements in adherence and that it was now time that additional efforts be directed towards developing and testing innovative approaches to assist patients to follow treatment prescriptions.

The causes of non-adherence

Some of the earliest studies investigated the hypothesis that non-adherence was caused by a lack of knowledge on the patients' part. This very rational view is appealing and suggests that explanations are all that is needed. The research shows that lack of knowledge does not account for poor compliance, and neither is compliance associated with social class, although social class differences between the doctor and the patient (particularly differences in education) may account for many communication difficulties (Becker and Maiman 1975).

Marshall Becker (1982) also helpfully demonstrated how a patient's experience of illness and medical care might conspire to reinforce his or her non-adherence. A patient may get well or not get well; and a patient may follow the recommended treatment plan or not, thus:

	Patient gets well	Patient does not get well
Patient complies	A	B
Patient does not comply	C	D

Patient A has been reinforced in his adherence, and patient D has been 'punished' for not following the advice given. But in the case of patient B, any one of a number of calamities may have occurred:

◆ an incorrect diagnosis may have been made

◆ inappropriate management may have been recommended

◆ efficacious medicines may have been prescribed but not in appropriate doses

◆ the patient may have tried to follow the instructions but got it wrong.

Patient B's efforts to follow the instructions will not be rewarded. Similarly, patient C would have been rewarded for not following the doctor's suggestions. In this way, adherence can be punished and non-adherence rewarded.

Adherence and the consultation

The way a consultation is conducted influences patient adherence. The style of consulting that works most effectively is one in which patients are fully involved in all aspects – including diagnosis and decisions about the management of the problem. It is a wonderful irony that, in order to increase patient adherence, doctors have to create a partnership of power with the patient in which the patient is the senior partner. However pushed for time the doctor may be, authoritarian consulting styles tend not to work. If the diagnosis and treatment are seen as the doctor's alone, then adherence is likely to be poor. If the diagnosis and treatment have been arrived at together, adherence is likely to increase.

Patients both prefer, and do better, when they are involved in the medical decision making process. David Smith *et al.* (1994), in a study of expressed consultation preferences using the Autonomy Preference Index, found that patients in the United Kingdom, the United States and Australia all expressed a clear preference for joint decision making rather than either delegating the decision to the doctor or deciding alone. Brody *et al.* (1989) demonstrated that involving patients in the decisions in the consultation leads to increased adherence afterwards.

Sherrie Kaplan and colleagues (1989) studied the effect of consultations not only on adherence but also on control of hypertension and diabetes. They found that

> ...poorer control of diabetes and hypertension at follow-up was associated with less patient control, less effective information seeking by, and less involvement of, the patient and less emotion/exchange of opinions by physician and patient during the baseline office visit

Consultations can make a significant difference both to adherence and to health. The consultations that make a difference involve patients in every aspect, encouraging questions and sharing decisions with the patients. This may be more uncomfortable for the physician but it improves health outcomes and reduces functional limitations.

Lassen (1991) used five criteria describing patient centred behaviours to assess consultations and predict adherence. These were that the doctor:

- explored the patient's expectations and ideas
- explained any advice
- gave reasons for any advice given
- checked the patient's views
- explored any obstacles to adherence

The difference between the rates of adherence in patients in those in whose consultations the criteria were fulfilled and those in which they were not was 44 per cent. If patient centred consulting were a drug with this magnitude of benefit, we would all wish to prescribe it.

Tailoring

Involvement is not the only factor that makes a difference. The other powerful factor is tailoring. By tailoring, we mean adapting the recommendations in the consultation to the unique circumstances of the patient. Standardizing recommendations and explanations may be tempting to a hard-pressed clinician, but it is counter-productive. Patients tend to disregard or minimize the significance of general explanations and advice. They pay more attention to, and follow through with, advice that is believed to be for them personally. The minimal conditions for tailoring appear to be that the patient feels the doctor knows him/her as a person, and explains the treatment decisions with this personal knowledge in mind (Smith *et al.* 1994).

Long-term outcomes

There is now a considerable body of evidence from a variety of settings that patient centred methods improve patients' health. In addition to the studies of Kaplan *et al.* (1989) reported above, Stewart (1995) reviewed 21 randomized controlled trials of physician–patient communication in which patient health was an outcome variable. The quality of the communication during history taking and discussion of the management plan positively affected patient health outcomes in 16 of the studies. These included emotional health, symptom resolution, function, physiological measures, and pain control.

Bass and colleagues (1986), in a study of 193 patients attending primary care physicians for common non-respiratory tract infections, found that agreement between physician and patient about the nature of the problem predicted resolution of the patient's symptom at one month, after controlling for demographic, psychological and social variables.

Lesley Fallowfield *et al.* (1990) studied a cohort of women with breast cancer treated by three groups of surgeons, one whose policy favoured mastectomy, a second who favoured breast conservation, and a third who offered a choice of treatment. There was considerable psychiatric morbidity post-operatively at 3 and 12 months after treatment in all three groups, and no differences between the patients who had had a mastectomy and those that had not. However, the patients treated by the surgeons whose policy was to offer the patient a choice, including those who for clinical reasons in fact had no choice, had significantly reduced anxiety and depression compared to the other two groups.

Litigation

One long-term outcome of health care that has become of increasing concern to doctors since the early 1980s, has been the patient (or relative) making a complaint or embarking on litigation. Strangely, not all adverse events result in a suit, and not all suits involve adverse events. In an attempt to elucidate the reasons why some patients choose to sue, Beckman *et al.* (1994) reviewed the statements made by plaintiffs in 45 malpractice suits against one metropolitan medical centre in New York. In answer to the question 'Why are you suing?' problematic relationships were identified in 71 per cent of the depositions. The themes that emerged were unavailability (32%), devaluing the views of patients or relatives (29%), poor delivery of information (26%), and failing to understand the patient or family perspective (13%). The annual reports of the medical defence and protection societies in the United Kingdom also contain frequent reports of communication failures as the precipitant of complaints and litigation.

Summary: a moral dilemma?

1. In order to be considered effective, consultations have to achieve tasks that lead to desirable outcomes. The most desirable long-term outcome is a positive change in the patient's health. This depends on sound diagnosis and appropriate actions taken to address the presenting problem. Non-adherence is an intermediate outcome that can render the consultation ineffective.

2. Yet some argue that adherence is not necessarily a good thing. Medical fallibility leads to errors and non-adherence may be justifiable on these grounds. There is also the matter of individual freedom and responsibility. Patients have to suffer the consequences of their decisions and so, arguably, they should be encouraged to take the decisions themselves when they are able to do so.

These arguments potentially pose a dilemma. Consultations could be conducted so as to maximize adherence or maximize patient choice. Fortunately, the evidence suggests that the same consulting style maximizes both simultaneously. Consultations that maximize choice (and involvement in the consultation) also increase the probability that patients will follow through with the plan created in the consultation. These consultations put the patient in greater control and contribute to their understanding of their health so that they are more able to make well-informed decisions.

5 Understanding the doctor

Introduction

There is little published research on the doctor's side of the cycle of care, though a great deal has been written about doctors in general, and about their relationship with patients. Society abounds with stereotypes, TV soap-operas, and popular reading overflow with doctors in all shapes and guises.

Curiously, patients do not seem to go to great lengths to seek out specific doctors and most patients seem to be relatively contented with their own doctors. Patients seem to rationalize that the sort of doctor they want is the sort of doctor they have (Fitton and Acheson 1979). Two poems may illustrate the patient's dilemma over the diversity of doctors. The first was WH Auden's view of the sort of physician he would want, and the second is Marie Campkin's chilling modern response:

Auden:

> Give me a doctor partridge plump,
> Short in the leg and broad in the rump,
> An endomorph with gentle hands,
> Who'll never make absurd demands
> That I abandon all my vices,
> Or pull a long face in a crisis,
> But with a twinkle in his eye,
> Will tell me that I have to die.

Campkin:

> Give me a doctor underweight,
> Computerised and up to date.
> A businessman who understands
> Accountancy and target bands.
> Who demonstrates sincere devotion
> To audit and to health promotion-
> But when my outlook's for the worse
> Refers me to the practice nurse.

Whereas in the last chapter we described, in detail, the patient's side of the cycle of care, similar evidence about the doctor's beliefs and understanding and about the outcomes for the doctor is not so easy to find. There has been much written about the 'burn out' of doctors and doctors' stress but this has not been related to the effect of individual consultations. In Chapter 3, we discussed the professional and societal context of the consultation and the general and specific ethical issues that affect it, yet the effect of these factors on specific consultations is relatively unknown.

In this chapter we will try to piece together the doctor's cycle. We will seek to understand the doctor: what motivates or demotivates, and what maintains or changes a doctor's consulting style. This will give some clues as to how most doctors may be effectively trained and further developed. We will also identify issues that need further research. We will draw on research evidence where it exists, and on our collective experience of medical care where the research is thin or absent.

Like a patient, the doctor comes to a consultation with many pre-determined attitudes, values and beliefs, which have emerged over years of training and experience. Other influences emerge closer to the consultation itself such as mood, tiredness, and enthusiasm for the current workload. Still others are related to the specific patient who is to be seen next.

All these factors affect the doctor's behaviour in a consultation and can make the consultation more or less effective for both the doctor and the patient. After a particular consultation the doctor, like the patient, experiences immediate and intermediate outcomes that can play a significant part in influencing subsequent consultations with that particular patient and others.

The doctor's understanding

The same distinctions hold for doctors as for patients (see Chapter 4). There are cognitive factors (knowledge, ideas and beliefs), emotional factors (feelings and concerns), and behavioural factors (skills and coping mechanisms).

Cognitive factors

Doctors' knowledge and understanding

In medical school, doctors learn about diseases and techniques to diagnose and treat them. Doctors are taught pattern recognition and how to come to a diagnosis by taking a history and by interpreting tests, signs, and symptoms. This very intense examination-based form of teaching produces people who gain a lot of knowledge 'by rote' and who sometimes fail to understand the principles and themes in the lessons. There is so much knowledge that it is difficult, if not impossible, to encompass it all. Without due care in the teaching of medicine, doctors can lose their understanding of people and what makes them tick just as they seem to become less skilled in communication.

Good doctors use their consultations with their patients to *increase* their knowledge, not merely to apply it. Over time, many hone their skills, and improve their understanding of illness, of people and also, importantly, of themselves. They draw all these strands together in the consultation and are increasingly at ease with both their knowledge and the gaps in their knowledge.

The application of knowledge to an individual patient is essential for effective care. Doctors must learn prioritization, how to sift information and to recognize meaning. A major problem facing the profession is consistency of the application of the doctor's knowledge. Often the same doctor prescribes different treatments for virtually identical ailments and patients are often bewildered by conflicting advice, not just from different doctors but often from the same doctor on different days. In an important study, Norwegian researchers sent two elderly women, pretending to have angina, in standardized presentation to 23 Trondheim GPs. They found that the same doctor did different things to identical patients on different occasions (Rethans and Saebu 1997).

Knowledge is often taught to doctors in the form of models, the most obvious in this context being 'the medical model', which is a disease-based way of looking at people's problems. How well doctors maintain and update their knowledge is a worry currently taxing many professional bodies. The movement from continuing medical education (CME), that had a great emphasis on updating of medical facts, to Continuing Professional Development (CPD) places the focus on the application of knowledge in the workplace and improving patient care. How informed the doctor is and how capable they are of applying that knowledge plays a major part in the effectiveness of the consultation.

Values, beliefs, and attitudes

On many issues doctors are not neutral. Like patients, they too have views that precede and pervade their consultations. Values, beliefs, and attitudes are words that refer to these influences on the consultation. Further, there is a continuum suggested by them. Values carry the greatest moral weight and are more permanent. Beliefs and attitudes carry slightly less force and are rather more susceptible to change.

Doctors' values, beliefs, and attitudes range over the full spectrum of medical care. They are often discussed in the context of such weighty issues as euthanasia and termination of pregnancy, but they apply equally well to whether or not patients should be prescribed antibiotics. The operative word here is 'should', since all these views carry a moral imperative about which the doctor may be more or less willing to compromise.

A few simple examples illustrate the point with respect to values and beliefs:

1. If the doctor is an atheist, she is less likely to suggest a dying patient to seek solace in God.

2. If he believes in the total sanctity of human life, the doctor will seldom recommend a termination of pregnancy or get involved in discussions about euthanasia.

3. If she believes that it is better for patients that they are protected from the whole truth in serious illness, then she will withhold information.

4. If her belief is that the major job of a doctor is to diagnose serious disease, then patients' worries and problems are seen by her as trivial.

5. If he believes that the patient's ideas and concerns are important then, the doctor will seek them out, and so on.

The debate about the role of the doctor in prevention and the early diagnosis of disease highlights that there are wide differences between doctors. Some would advocate a very pro-active role with multiple screening and active intervention in patients' lives. Others feel that screening for disease and advising about life style is an invasion of the patient's privacy and is not part of the doctor's job. Most doctors would fall somewhere in between.

The key point here is awareness. Doctors who remain unaware of the influence of their values on their work are more likely to impose them unwittingly on their patients. Doctors who are aware of their biases can take them into account. All doctors, moreover, have to remain sensitive to the needs of the patient and to recognize when a retreat from the doctor's personal convictions would be appropriate in the interests of the good care of a particular patient.

Skills and experience

Doctors have a wide variety of skills and experience that they bring to the consultation. There are medical skills such as the use of the opthalmascope, or joint injection; consultation skills such as exploring beliefs about health and illness; and personal skills such as making people feel at ease. These skills have been developed over many years both in formal medical training and in broader experience in life.

Many would expect that knowledge, attitudes, and beliefs directly influence behaviour, and that skills are simply recruited to achieve objectives. The matter is not as simple as that, however, and skills can powerfully affect attitudes and beliefs in the longer term. Few doctors, for example, will sustain a belief about how to consult with patients if they feel unable to demonstrate such an approach within the time and resources available to them in the consultation. Instead, they invent self-sustaining attitudes and beliefs that justify how they consult. This reaction is entirely human and protects their self-esteem. When we discuss the teaching of effective consulting skills we will come back to this relationship between the doctor's values and attitudes on the one hand, and his/her consultation behaviour on the other.

Emotional factors

Doctors are as affected by emotional factors in their work as is any other professional, but these factors are often ignored or denied by medical educators. The part these factors play in the consultation is complex. The place of doctors' self esteem, fears, anxieties, and confidence is thinly researched, but often discussed by doctors and patients alike.

How doctors feel affects how they consult. It is obvious that consulting is likely to be more effective when the doctor is in good physical health, but many doctors, driven by inner goals, soldier on when they are sick long after they should. Emotional health is subtler and more insidious. Doctors have a very high incidence of alcoholism, depressive illness, and chronic stress disorders. These illnesses drastically limit the doctor's ability to consult but many force themselves to carry on, inappropriately, rarely seeking help from colleagues, as this is perceived as a sign of weakness. Fortunately, there are signs that the profession, and its professional organizations, are beginning to wake up to the emotional needs of doctors. In the United Kingdom, for example, doctors in distress can seek help from a national help-line, and the professional bodies are funding the investigation and treatment of medical stress.

Many doctors consult in such a way as to protect their emotional health. Emotional involvement with patients can increase the emotional strain. When patients die with whom the doctor is close, it hurts. When several patients die with whom the doctor is close, it hurts a lot. In a study of palliative care physicians (Ford et al. 1996) the amount of empathy and social involvement was almost nil in otherwise very efficient and thorough medical encounters. This is probably a defence mechanism adopted by many doctors in all specialities. For doctors facing a long career of emotional bruising, it is not surprising that many develop closed and protective styles of communication. Yet with support and understanding, doctors can change their consultations to be more open and sharing, retaining their humanity without damaging consequences.

Temperament makes a difference to most spheres of activity. Whether one is optimistic or pessimistic is, to some extent, an act of will. The ability to maintain positive emotions is also a personality characteristic associated with extraversion. There is little published research about the effects of these characteristics on consulting, but it is a reasonable hypothesis that a doctor's positive or negative orientation will influence his or her patients.

Behavioural factors

Doctors' style

By style we mean the doctor's characteristic approach to consultations that is largely consistent over time. Most doctors believe that their behaviour varies significantly from patient to patient. Byrne and Long (1976), however, after studying a very large number of consultations from a broad range of doctors, concluded that doctors' style varied little from consultation to consultation. They even claimed, 'once a doctor has developed their style there is a danger that it becomes a prison in which they are forced to work'. A doctor's style can also be the basis of his/her coping mechanism for the purposes of self-protection. The more insight and supportive feedback about these factors the doctor receives, the more likely he/she is to develop a style that is effective for the patients and for him/herself.

The style of a doctor is an amalgam of learned factors such as habits, skills, attitudes, and beliefs. Byrne and Long (1976) described a spectrum of consulting styles that ranged from doctor-centred to patient-centred but found that style was relatively fixed in their sample of mature doctors. They found that their doctors tended to do similar things in consultations with minimal regard to the patient and the complaint. More recent evidence suggests that this is not the case for doctors in training. Evidence from the video component of the UK's Royal College of General Practitioners (RCGP) membership examination suggests that style is still quite variable and erratic at this relatively early stage in a doctor's career (Tate *et al.* 1999).

Roter *et al.* (1997) identified four styles in practising US doctors:

(1) *Paternalism*: the doctor-centred style;

(2) *Consumerism*: in which the patient is firmly in the driving seat;

(3) *Default or laissez-faire*: in which neither party takes responsibility and produces a formless and aimless consultation;

(4) *Mutuality*: where both the doctor and the patient are involved, patient preferences are actively sought and compared with the doctor's. The whole process is one of negotiation.

Mutuality is the process we advocate and is relatively rare in the United Kingdom. Tuckett *et al.* (1985) found that detailed explanations were sparse in British General Practice consultations. They found that what they called 'reactive explanations', in which the doctor explained in response to a patient's ideas or beliefs, occurred in fewer than one in 10 consultations. Real patient involvement in the decision making process occurred in fewer than one in 100 consultations. Recent analysis of over 1000 young family doctors who had submitted videotaped consultations for the RCGP membership examination found only 8 out of 100 able to demonstrate mutuality in three out of five selected consultations, even when they knew that the examination criteria would favour a mutual style.

Arguably, patients' style and locus of control should influence doctors' behaviour in the consultation, but empirical evidence of this occurring is hard to find. Patients who want to be involved may find it hard to be, but this area needs more research. Medical education needs to equip doctors with a broad repertoire of consulting skills to enable them to deal effectively with a broad range of patients and a broad range of needs.

Style and gender

There is increasing evidence that the communication style of doctors is not related to gender. This has been demonstrated in the RCGP membership examination (Tate *et al.* 1999) and by Skelton and Hobbs (1999). Male doctors, by contrast, have hitherto been caricatured as less involving than their female counterparts. In fact, it appears that effective communication in the consultation needs to be learned and can be learned equally well by men and women.

The consultation's immediate context

Consultations have two different types of immediate influence: those that are unrelated to the specific patient, and those that are patient-related.

Factors unrelated to the patient

There are at least three different types of immediate, non-patient-related influences on a consultation. These include the physical environment, the managerial arrangements in the practice, and the doctor's mood and health.

The physical environment

The buildings and equipment of a doctor's office can exert an influence on how he or she works with patients. It may be expected that a clean, well-decorated building with adequate space in which to practise medicine can elevate the mood of patient and doctor alike. Whereas, if the office is dingy, uncomfortable, inadequately private, and poorly equipped, the standard of care offered is placed at risk. Good care is not impossible to provide under adverse circumstances, but more difficult to sustain.

The managerial arrangements

A lengthy wait when a doctor is running late can put the doctor under pressure. The same wait can sufficiently irritate both doctor and patient to make it difficult to establish rapport in the consultation. Unrealistic appointment schedules are common causes of difficulties between doctors and patients.

The results are that the doctor feels and appears to be rushed to the detriment of the consultation. Good medical care requires a certain amount of time. It may be extremely difficult to look after patients well if time is too short, though many would want to debate how long is 'enough'. We want to argue here that feeling under pressure further exacerbates any actual shortage of time.

Good medical care also requires concentration. If the consultation is frequently interrupted, whether by ringing phones or colleagues coming in and out of the doctor's office, the communication process is hindered. Good records are an additional element of good medical care, but their maintenance during the consultation can become an impediment. Similarly, poorly organized records in which notes, letters, and test results are missing or hard to find, cause irritation to the doctor and distress to the patient.

As computers become more common in the consulting room, the same issues arise. It is very easy for the computer to distract the doctor from concentrating on the patient and his/her problem. The doctor needs to be aware of this potential and manage the transitions between patient and computer, without detriment to the patient or the consultation process. Those who wish to focus on their patients may find the computer a significant hindrance.

The doctor's mood and health

The doctor may be having a good or bad day emotionally for many reasons. It matters little whether the cause is to be found in the medical practice, at home, or elsewhere. Mood has an influence on the consultation and strongly negative moods can cause serious problems for doctor and patient. Experienced and strong-minded professionals can control this effect to some extent but the doctor needs to be able to remain sensitive to emotions in order to be effective. On some days, pressures are particularly strong. In these circumstances, the doctor concentrates on just getting through the day, cutting responses to a minimum, and avoiding involvement.

Ill-health presents the doctor with a dilemma. A doctor with concern for his or her colleagues will not want to let them down or cause them undue pressure. A stoical doctor may minimize his/her ill-health and its effects. A mistrustful doctor may not believe that his/her patients will be well treated by colleagues. In these cases, doctors may work when their effectiveness is reduced. By contrast, doctors whose enthusiasm has waned may seek any acceptable excuse not to work, and a doctor with concern not to infect already sick patients may also stay away from the office.

Roger Neighbour, in his book The Inner Consultation (1987), introduced the concept of 'housekeeping', to describe the need for doctors to look after their own mental and physical well being, especially in their particular profession (see Chapter 8). Patients affect the doctor's emotions. Doctors vary in the level of emotional involvement they seek or can cope with, but Michael Balint pointed out that sad patients (inevitably) make doctors sad, and doctors deal continually in sadness, ill health, lost hopes, and death.

Factors that are patient-related

Individual patients can produce an emotional reaction in the doctor that is either positive or negative. These emotions can spill over into subsequent consultations with that patient and affect how the doctor manages that consultation.

Some patients cheer us up, most are neutral emotionally, and some produce profoundly gloomy feelings. Naturally, patients will not affect all doctors in the same way.

O'Dowd coined the term *heart-sink* (O'Dowd 1988) and, though the term has pejorative implications, it soon became part of medical language. The original article was not particularly negative about the patients that caused these emotions: it recognized that different doctors have different heart-sink perceptions and that recognizing those emotions can have a positive view on the management of those patients.

The question that must concern us is: how significant are negative emotions about patients to the consultation process? Some authors have defined the characteristic of heart-sink to be doctors feeling helpless in the face of those patients who seek salvation for psychological, social, and spiritual problems by bio-medical means (Butler and Evans 1999). The 'heart-sink' phenomenon may be a symptom of tension within the philosophical foundations of not only General Practice but also the whole bio-medical model of medical care.

Mathers *et al.* (1995) thought there was an average of six heart-sink patients per UK GP with a range of 1–50. This remarkable range may of course point not so much to the distribution of the patients but to the attitudinal differences between the doctors. Schwenk (1987) demonstrated that difficult doctor–patient relationships were associated with two to three times higher rates of investigations and referrals. Balint (1957), and subsequent authors writing in the Balint tradition, emphasize that greater understanding of the patients that cause the doctor problems can often help to develop a management plan and diminish the negative emotions that the doctor might have about the patient.

The consultation itself

The doctor enters into any consultation with many direct and indirect influences already having their effect. Patterns are set, a definite hypothesis may already be made, and firm management decisions may be taken before the patient even enters the room. The awareness and insight of the doctor about these issues can substantially modify their effect on the consultation. To those involved in teaching doctors and other health care professionals, sensitivity to these issues can be the key to bringing about improvement in consulting effectiveness.

Outcomes for the doctor

In Chapter 4, we described outcomes for patients with reference to the time that elapsed between the consultation and the outcome. In this way we described immediate, intermediate, and long-term outcomes for patients. Here we take a similar approach to outcomes for the doctor though with much less direct empirical evidence upon which to draw.

Immediate outcomes: rewards and punishments

Rewards

The sheer weight of the workload may cause some doctors to take some pleasure that a consultation has merely ended. This is negative reinforcement to those with a behaviourist orientation: the removal of a noxious stimulus. More frequently, doctors will draw significant satisfaction from a diagnosis made, a problem well-managed, an encounter with a friendly and (usually) grateful patient, and the opportunity to make a difference to someone's life, family, and/or health.

Punishments

Other immediate outcomes can be punishing. The doctor may have been unable to cope with the patient's problem. The patient may have been dissatisfied with the consultation. The doctor may have felt impotent to help and/or transfer responsibility back to the patient. The relationship with the patient may have been negative. The effects of poor practice management may also have taken their toll, such as running late, feeling rushed, and the frequency of interruptions.

Intermediate outcome: feedback

The feedback doctors get from their patients is haphazard and unsystematic. The doctor cannot assume that compliments are the result of a job well done, or that anger implies failure. The whole situation is much more complex than that. Certainly, negative feedback, such as receiving a formal complaint, can seem overwhelming, and a malpractice accusation can be devastating. Frequently, doctors receive a series of mild statements of gratitude and, though the reason for the gratitude may be far from clearly understood, the feedback can be deceptive. Typically, there is little or no feedback either within or subsequent to a consultation and the doctor makes of that what he or she will: good or bad.

More systematic feedback from patients can be elicited by asking for it. At follow-up consultations, information can be sought not only about the management of the problem but also about the consultation process. Thoughts can be ascertained about the advice given and the amount of retained knowledge; feelings after the last consultation of satisfaction/dissatisfaction can be described, and the extent of the patient's compliance with medication or advice can be reported. There are also more formal ways of seeking feedback from patients: questionnaires, interviews, or focus groups. These will be covered in more detail in a later chapter.

A direct parallel to the patient's experience also exists. The doctor will observe the effect of his/her practice on the patients' health and draw conclusions from it:

	Patient gets well	Patient does not get well
Doctor complies with professional protocols	A	B
Doctor ignores professional protocols	C	D

The doctor could draw conclusions from experience with patients A and D that recommended protocols are effective. Whereas experience with patients B and D could shake the doctor's faith in the protocols.

Given the variety of influences on whether or not patients get well, this feedback is extremely unreliable. It is essentially superstitious: the associations inferred between the doctor's behaviour and its consequences for the patient are not necessarily causal. Yet causal conclusions tend to be drawn from this flimsy evidence in the name of clinical experience when the full evidence base is ignored or when the doctor insulates him/herself from true peer review.

Longer-term outcomes

When a doctor's professional experience is compared with that of many other professions, most of Abraham Maslow's hierarchy of needs are met in most circumstances (Maslow 1970). There is no concern about physiological needs (food and shelter) or safety needs (fear of danger and job insecurity) in the minds of most doctors. It is the higher needs that can cause satisfaction or dissatisfaction—those of belonging (feeling wanted), autonomy (being in control of ones life), and self-actualization (having a feeling of self worth). There are opportunities to fulfil all these needs in medical practice depending on the doctor's attitudes to, perceptions of, and experience of the rewards and punishments.

In the short-term, satisfaction may be derived from a good clinical performance, a clever diagnosis, perhaps the revealing of distress by touch and use of silence. In the longer-term, job satisfaction may depend on the doctor's values. For some, the intellectual detective work of medical encounters is the spur and the reward. For others, job satisfaction is gained from reversing the medical model and un-organizing symptoms, trying to give the responsibility for minor malaise back to patients and not creating illness and disease out of the problems of daily living. For most, there are rewards in feeling skilful, and in being trusted, respected and valued.

The personal relationship between doctor and patient may also contribute to longer-term job satisfaction. Some doctors prefer to adopt an authoritarian style and to have patients who are deferential. Others are much happier with an adult, sharing relationship. Many doctors want to be liked, others find innocent flirtation engaging and some even use prescriptions like presents to curry favour. Grateful patients can also flatter the doctor's ego, while others prefer a more distant relationship with their patients finding familiarity uncomfortable.

The general conclusion we want to draw is that understanding the doctor is a task for the doctor him/herself. Awareness of the doctor's values and style, strengths, and limitations allows these factors to be taken into account. Awareness of the doctor's needs allows them to be met. Respect for the doctor's needs makes meeting them within the practice more likely.

Summary

1. Doctors' behaviour in consultations varies widely between doctors.

2. The variation in doctors' behaviour in consultations is based in part on the doctor's 'understanding' that is influenced by cognitive, emotional, and other behavioural factors.

3. The doctor's behaviour is also influenced by a variety of other immediate contextual factors, some of which are patient-related.

4. Outcomes for the doctor can be seen in terms of perceived rewards and punishments that accumulate to determine the doctor's job satisfaction.

5. Effective feedback for doctors is hard to come by and needs to be actively sought from patients and peers.

6. It is important to maintain the doctor's mental and physical health for the sake of both parties.

6 Understanding the consultation

In the previous chapters we have considered how the individual consultation should be seen as part of a cycle of care, with inputs from both the patient and the doctor, outcomes that can be short, intermediate, or long term. We have also described how the consultation is influenced by the social and ethical contexts in which the medical care is taking place. We are now in a position to consider what actually takes place in the consultation between the patient and the doctor.

There are a large number of approaches, which describe different aspects of the consultation. They vary in the way that they have been developed and in their purpose. Some have an evidence base, while others are derived from theoretical considerations. Some have been used for developmental or descriptive studies, or for teaching, while others are based on studies that link aspects of the consultation to outcomes. Most are based on a model of a single medical interview in which a patient presents with a problem, which is then diagnosed and managed, rather than on a series of consultations in which the relationship and the content develop over time. Many seek to describe the content of a medical interview in any setting rather than particularly in primary care.

In this chapter, we will not attempt a comprehensive review of the literature but will describe those contributions that have influenced our thinking. We will then propose a unifying framework that incorporates these ideas and encapsulates our approach to analysing and teaching the consultation.

Describing the consultation

Some approaches have started from the verbal and non-verbal communication that can be observed, which leads to descriptions of behaviours and skills. Others, notably those based on the work of Michael Balint (1957), started with the participants' descriptions of their current thoughts and feelings about the consultation which led to the development of insights into their intentions, their thoughts, and feelings during the consultation, and the nature of the relationship between the doctor, the patient, and the illness.

Many people have found the distinction between tasks, strategies, and skills a helpful starting point in understanding the consultation.

1. *Tasks* describe what is to be achieved in the consultation, or in a phase of the consultation. They are statements of intent derived from the needs of the patient and the purposes or aims of the doctor.

2. *Strategies* are the plans or approaches that the doctor uses to achieve those tasks. Examples of strategies that can be used to achieve tasks include:

    (a) clinical reasoning and hypothesis testing to make a diagnosis;

    (b) reacting to and developing the patients' ideas to share understanding;

    (c) negotiation and goal setting to achieve behaviour change.

3. In contrast *skills* are purposeful and clearly observable behaviours and have therefore been used extensively as the basis for both teaching and research. A meta-analysis of over 60 papers correlated aspects of behaviour in the consultation with the outcomes of memory, satisfaction, and compliance (Roter and Hall 1989). Teaching programmes have sometimes selected skills on the evidence that links them to favourable outcomes.

This approach however has substantial limitations. It is possible that there are confounding variables such as the characteristics of the patients or their problems, that leads both to the variations in behaviour in the consultation and in subsequent outcome. Second, the correlations in most of the studies reviewed by Roter are in fact quite small and fail to explain the majority of the variation of outcome. Finally, the value of satisfaction as an outcome has been questioned in the light of other evidence that shows that approaches that are less directive and encourage patient involvement may threaten immediate satisfaction but can result in improved long-term health of the patient (Greenfield *et al.* 1985). In our experience, teaching skills without discussing and agreeing their purpose also runs the risk of being perceived as stereotyping by the learners and leads to resistance.

The principal advantage of basing teaching on tasks is that it enables a clear statement about the purposes of the consultation, which can be discussed and negotiated. These tasks can be derived from the needs of patients, the aims of the doctor, the desired outcomes, and the evidence that links them. This approach also recognizes that individual doctors use a variety of approaches and skills to achieve the same tasks. It also enables teachers to take a diagnostic approach with learners by considering the extent to which tasks are achieved, and then helping the learner develop those skills and strategies that will help them to increase their effectiveness. The principal limitation of focusing on tasks is that the feelings of the patient and doctor can be relatively neglected.

Descriptions based on tasks

There have been several consultation models based on tasks. We will describe seven here.

The tasks that we described in 1984 were similar to those described by The Department of Family Practice in London, Ontario (Levenstein *et al.* 1986). The Ontario group described a medical interview as exploring two agendas: the doctor's relatedness to the symptoms and disease, and the patients' including their concerns, fears, and illness experience, and then integrating these two

Box 6.1 **The patient-centred clinical method**

1. Exploring both the disease and the illness experience
   (a) Differential diagnosis
   (b) Dimensions of illness (ideas, feelings, expectations, and effects)
2. Understanding the whole person
   (a) The person (life history and personal development)
   (b) The context
3. Finding common ground regarding management
   (a) Problems and priorities
   (b) Goals of treatment
   (c) Roles of doctor and patient in management
4. Incorporating prevention and health promotion
   (a) Health enhancement
   (b) Risk reduction
   (c) Early detection of disease
   (d) Ameliorating effects of disease
5. Enhancing the doctor–patient relationship
   (a) Characteristics of the therapeutic relationship
   (b) Sharing power
   (c) Caring and healing relationship
   (d) Self-awareness
   (e) Transference and counter-transference
6. Being realistic
   (a) Time
   (b) Resources
   (c) Team building.

agendas. They have since described six interactive components in such a consultation, which share many of the characteristics of our tasks (Box 6.1).

In 1995, they published their book Patient-Centred Medicine (Stewart *et al.* 1995) describing the development of these concepts and ways in which they can be taught and evaluated, and the research evidence that supported them. They worked independently over the same period as our group in Oxford, but both are very happy to acknowledge the large amount of common ground there is between us. Their book is an impressive account of a coherent body of research and teaching development, which has been very influential internationally.

Cohen-Cole (1991) described three functions that take place in the medical interview:

(1)   gathering data to understand the patient;

(2)   building rapport and responding to patients' emotions;

(3)   education, negotiation, and motivation.

They also listed the basic skills required to achieve each of these fairly broad functions, and a nine-session model course to teach them. Variations of this approach have been adopted by many medical schools in the United States.

Roger Neighbour in *The Inner Consultation* (1987) describes five 'check-points' in the journey through a consultation:

(1)   connecting with the patient;

(2)   summarizing his understanding of the patient's problems;

(3)   handing over decisions and management;

(4)   'safety netting' to manage uncertainty and to avoid being caught by unexpected developments;

(5)   housekeeping, the doctor taking care of himself or herself to manage the stresses of clinical practice.

The Calgary-Cambridge observation guide (Kurtz and Silverman 1996) is based on five tasks:

(1)   initiating the session;

(2)   gathering information;

(3)   building the relationship;

(4)   explanation and planning;

(5)   closing the session.

They also described an expanded framework of skills, which provide further details of the steps to be achieved within each consultation.

More recently, Mead and Bower (2000) reviewed the literature and identified five conceptual dimensions of patient-centredness. These were:

(1)   A *biopsychosocial* perspective, expanding the scope of the consultation to include the social and psychological dimensions of health;

(2)   the '*patient-as-person*', understanding the individual's experience of illness;

(3)   sharing power and responsibility in the consultation;

(4)   *the therapeutic alliance*, recognizing that the relationship is not just about management but has therapeutic potential. This idea is similar to Michael Balint's idea of 'the drug *Doctor*';

(5)   *the doctor-as-person*, considering the contribution that the individual doctor makes to the relationship.

Bensing (2000) suggested that the concept of 'Patient-centredness' could be clarified by contrasting it to both disease- and doctor-centred care. The characteristics of patient-centredness are therefore:

(1) concern for the whole person rather than just their disease;

(2) the patient's involvement in controlling the consultation and setting the agenda;

(3) patients' expectations and power to make decisions.

Greater attention has also been given to what Elwyn, Edwards, and Kinnersley (1999) described as 'The neglected second half of the consultation' in which decisions are made about management. Discussions have included the ethical issues of the respect for patient autonomy and the right to make or to share decisions. They have also included the practical problems of sharing information, particularly about risk, and the process of decision-making. These discussions are taking place currently in the context of growing patient expectations of information and involvement, and the explosion in information technology.

The challenge is to bring all these concepts together in a coherent statement that does not lose its richness and complexity, but is also sufficiently clear to be of value in teaching and practice.

The tasks

The rest of the chapter will describe the consultation based on a revised set of tasks that contribute to an effective consultation, and consider which strategies and skills can be used to achieve them.

Task 1

To understand the reasons for the patient's attendance, including:

(1) *The patient's problem*:
  (a) *its nature and history*
  (b) *its aetiology*
  (c) *its effects.*

(2) *The patient's perspective*:
  (a) *their personal and social circumstances*
  (b) *their ideas and values about health*
  (c) *their ideas about the problem, its causes and its management*
  (d) *their concerns about the problem and its implications*
  (e) *their expectations for information, involvement, and care.*

Patients come with 'problems' rather than diseases and the task is to understand these problems, their *nature* and *history* and their *causes*, so that management can be directed whenever possible at causes rather than just effects.

This task also includes understanding the whole of the patient's *illness experience*, including the *effects* that the problems may be having on the patient's life, as well as on the patient's emotional responses. These may be both part of the problem and part of the reasons for consulting, and understanding them are clearly an important part of the consultation.

We have found it helpful to consider *ideas, concerns*, and *expectations* as conceptually distinct items. As has been described more fully in Chapter 4, each individual patient will have complex and varied ideas and beliefs both about health and illness in general, and about his or her own particular problems and its management. Establishing what these are enables the doctor to tailor the information they offer both to the patient's ideas and to the ways that they express them. Ideas reflect the patient's health understanding, and contain views specific to the problem and general attitudes to health, illness, treatments, and doctors.

Illnesses also have meanings and implications for patients that can generate *concerns*. Establishing what these are enables the doctor to offer appropriate reassurance, empathy, or support. There is good evidence that addressing patients' concerns is also therapeutic.

Most consultations include some decisions about investigations, treatment, and management. Patients will sometimes go to see a doctor with *expectations* about what these decisions will be. Establishing the patient's expectations allows the doctor either to meet or discuss them. Patients will also vary in the extent to which they expect to be informed and involved in decisions about their care. The evidence reviewed in earlier chapters indicates that while the preference of the majority is for shared decision making, this will vary with the nature of the problem, and the doctor needs to establish the preference of each individual in each case.

Since the first book there has been an increased emphasis on the patient's agenda, although this was part of the original Byrne and Long (1976) description. Agendas fulfil a similar role to expectations in that each is purposeful and determine the preferred course of the consultation. It is the combination of the concerns and expectations that most influence the decision to consult. The crucial point about agendas is that they are often concealed, because of fear, embarrassment, or uncertainty. It would seem self-evident that understanding why the patient has consulted is the essential first task in any consultation, and indeed Byrne and Long found that failure to do so was the commonest cause of dysfunctional consultations.

To consider appropriate strategies it is necessary to concentrate on the word '*understand*' in the first task. Understanding is not easy and human beings are unique. The first strategy is to create a state of mind that wants to know about the patient. Doctors need to be curious and, with curiosity, several other useful strategies fall into place. There is a tendency then to listen and not to talk. There is evidence that listening and not interrupting early in encounters allows a greater revelation of the patient's narrative (Beckman and Frankel 1984).

Another effective strategy is to attempt to identify oneself with the patient, and so comprehend them better. This is the Oxford Dictionary definition of empathy. Anthropologists have suggested that all patients everywhere ask themselves several questions before making a medical visit. What could be wrong? Why has it happened? Why to me? Why now? What will happen? The doctor can anticipate these issues will be relevant for most patients but not in all consultations. A good strategy is to listen, and then feed back to demonstrate empathy.

Curiosity, listening, and empathy will go a long way to eliciting the patient's perspective but medical care requires strategies and skills in addition. There is an inherent conflict here between traditional medical teaching which concentrates on the disease, and a person-centred approach. Medical history taking is a comprehensive, doctor-centred model designed primarily for pattern recognition of illness. But it is ill-suited to most medical encounters because of time constraints and its lack of concern with the person. Nevertheless, doctors are trained to take a history with all that implies.

Taking a history is a method of controlling what the patient says. The medical model encourages doctors to take control of the interview and to chase symptoms with staccato, closed questions establishing data such as time, place, type, severity, and so on. This can be fun if it appeals to the Sherlock Holmes in all doctors and satisfies some clinical curiosity. Certainly most patients would prefer a bad communicator who got the serious diagnosis correct, to the good communicator who missed it.

Yet, the imperative enshrined in this first task is that doctors must learn both to diagnose *and* to communicate; it is nothing less than a new way of 'history taking'. It has become clear over the last twenty years that this is a complex task to achieve in its entirety, and that the strategies and skills required to discern the nature and history and the medical aetiology are of a different order from those required to elucidate the patient's perspective. It requires a sophisticated level of communication ability to synthesize the medical and biosocial models, and the full achievement of this task, while an ideal and a goal for medical personnel, will remain elusive in many encounters.

The following questions are good indicators of how well our first task has been achieved:

1. Do I know significantly more about the patient than before the consultation?

2. Was I curious?

3. Did I listen?

4. Did I explore the patient's ideas, concerns, expectations, and the effects of the problem?

5. Did I acknowledge the patient's viewpoint?

6. Did I make an acceptable working diagnosis?

Task 2

Taking into account the patient's perspective, to achieve a shared understanding:

(1) *about the problem;*

(2) *about the evidence and options for management.*

Patients want and expect to be told about their problem and its management in ways that they can remember and understand. Their satisfaction with the consultation is substantially influenced by the amount of information they are given. What is more, reduction of uncertainty is in itself therapeutic. Patients need to understand their condition and its treatment to enable them to manage it themselves more effectively, including the decision about when to consult again. Patients cannot participate in shared decision making about treatment unless they understand the options and their implications. In addition to these benefits for the patient, patients who are not fully informed about risks or side effects of treatment are more likely to sue (successfully) when they occur. Thus it is in the interests of both doctor and patient to ensure that a shared understanding is achieved.

David Tuckett described a consultation as a Meeting Between Experts, (Tuckett *et al*. 1985) with the aim of sharing each other's understanding. The process he described was 'reactive explanation' with the doctor using the patient's concepts, ideas and also their language so that the information fits in with their own explanatory models. Tuckett also found that in the 20 per cent of consultations after which the patient was unable to remember the key messages they had been given, the commonest reason was that the explanations of the doctor did not fit with the ideas the patient already had.

With the growth of Evidence Based Medicine there will be some consultations in which explanations are required about the risks and benefits of treatment, and this raises the question about how such explanations are framed. Understandings of the words *common, possible*, or *rare* can vary and the use of percentages or other figures may be interpreted in different ways. For example, patients are more likely to take a treatment if told that it will reduce their risk of another heart attack by a third than if they are told that it reduces their risk from 12 to 8 per cent. They are even less accepting if told that the number of patients needing to be treated to prevent one attack is 25. The important task is to convey such information in ways that are meaningful to the individual patient while not manipulating the message.

There is a growth in so-called motivational interviewing (Miller 1983), which is a methodology designed to help in those very difficult areas of addiction. The premise is that the doctor can help explore consequences and alternatives but it is the patient and only the patient who ultimately chooses what will be done. However, the recommended technique is often to 'spin' the options in such as a way as to get the patient to achieve the desired health outcome. In this case, the end justifies the means and is more Machiavellian than Motivational.

Most consultations involve uncertainty and we would argue that part of the task is to help patients understand and tolerate it rather than seek to protect them from it. We believe the underlying ethos must be of honesty, even when this means acknowledging the frailties of medical knowledge and predictions. Indeed, the medical profession has not done anyone any favours in the past by pretending that diagnoses can always be made, that screening will detect all abnormalities, and that treatments are risk free.

The question doctors must ask is not 'have I achieved a shared understanding?' but 'how do I know that I have?' This highlights the worrying results of recent research (Tate *et al.* 1999) that shows checking of understanding is very rare. In fact, only 6 per cent of specially selected consultations submitted for the Membership of the Royal College of General Practitioners (MRCGP) examination in the United Kingdom contained any real shared understanding or shared decision-making.

The reality is that this task usually comes immediately at the end of the diagnostic/examination phase of the consultation. However involved, the patient usually becomes passive and expectant waiting for the revelatory pronouncements of the doctor. What results is usually an explanation, which is a one way process, from doctor to patient. Sharing of understanding is a two way process and cannot occur unless the doctor understands the patient's perspective.

Doctors who are sharing understanding are also formulating management plans and strategies while talking and listening. The act of sharing understanding is intended to clarify, modify, and tailor the subsequent decision, making it more appropriate to the patient. Much of the effective sharing will be in the realm of wants, needs, fears, and beliefs. Unemotional logic is not the essence of general practice. Rather, shared understanding is achieved when the patient's knowledge and expectations are in line with the likely aetiology and management of the problem and its prognosis.

Task 3

To enable the patient to choose an appropriate action for each problem

(1) *consider options and implications;*
(2) *choose the most appropriate course of action.*

In the majority of consultations, decisions are made either explicitly or implicitly about management, and choices are being made between options ranging between doing nothing, self-care, prescription, or referral. The headline issue is whether these decisions are made by the doctor, the patient, or the two of them together. The underlying issue is how the decisions are made.

The classical decision-making process is to define the problem, define the options, consider the options, and decide. In a medical decision the options will have benefits but also risks, and differing probabilities of occurrence. An operation for knee replacement may have an 80 per cent chance of pain free mobility as its outcome, an 18 per cent risk of restricted mobility, and a 2 per cent mortality. These risks and benefits need to be presented in ways that the patient can understand (Edwards *et al.* 2002).

Different patients will place different weights on these outcomes. An elderly person who is housebound and in considerable pain may be much more willing to accept the risk of death than a younger person who is considering an operation because he cannot play golf. Patients may need help and time to consider the implications of the options for them before the decision is made.

Doctors do not only provide information but also offer their opinions, and many patients wish them to do so. Sharing the decision is about sharing information and opinions, and helping patients understand and consider the options, in a balanced way. Patients may initially state a preference for their doctor to make a decision, but when its implications are explained they are more likely to wish to be involved in the decision.

The main strategy required to complete this task successfully is one of effective negotiation, and it is to this end that skills training should be directed. The two principal areas of a doctor–patient negotiation are:

♦ recognizing and understanding the patient's perspective

♦ offering viable and understandable alternatives.

We recognize that patients may not wish to share in decisions; some are even panicked by the sudden change in the traditional doctor and patient roles. We are advocating that the normal state of general practice should be shared decision making, not that it must be achieved in all consultations irrespective of the patient's wishes. We acknowledge that there will be times when the doctor needs to decide, other times when informed decision making may be all that is attainable. Nevertheless, the aim is to share the decision-making process and this should become the norm.

The concept of shared decision making requires definition (Charles *et al.* 1997, 1999; Elwyn, Edwards, Gwyn, and Grol 1999) and new competencies to achieve it (Towle and Godolphin 1999).

A large proportion of consultations in primary care involve a prescription for short courses of treatment, many of which the patient did not expect or want (Britten *et al.* 2000). Discussion of these decisions can be brief and effective. For the patient to participate in more major decisions may require more time than is available in a single consultation. Offering patients time to consider and indicating other sources of information may be all that can be achieved in the short term.

. Increasing access to information has made shared decision making even more crucial. In our first book, we put this task before sharing understanding; we realize now that shared understanding is probably a prerequisite to shared decision making. All the tasks are important to achieve but the first five are clearly more sequential than at first we thought.

Task 4

To enable the patient to manage the problem:

(1) *discuss the patient's ability to take appropriate actions*;

(2) *agree doctor and patient actions and responsibilities*;

(3) *agree targets, monitoring, and follow up*.

The appropriateness of this task clearly depends on the nature of the proposed management. The role of the patient in the treatment of acute appendicitis is initially very passive, but post-operatively the speed of recovery can depend on the active participation of the patient. In primary care, management can include such measures as medication, psychological adjustment, or lifestyle change.

Involvement in medication is not an issue of adherence to doctors' orders. To take medication appropriately, to take the correct dose and to stop it when necessary for example, may require the patient to know what it is intended to do, to monitor progress, to recognize side effects and to respond to them. Patients with chronic diseases can become experts in their care. This requires both information and encouragement from the doctor.

Many psychological therapies aim to help patients recognize their symptoms and their causes, and to learn new behaviours and coping strategies. This requires a partnership between the patient and therapist, which enables the patient rather than the creation of dependence. While many illnesses have their root cause in unhealthy lifestyles, this task is not about victim blaming or convincing the patient that it is all their fault. It is about helping define what changes they would like to make, ensuring that they are able to do so, and providing appropriate support. It is clear however that when attempting to give health advice, it should be first established whether the patient wants it.

Whether the agreed action is a procedure, medication, therapy, or self-help and lifestyle change, the key issue is whether the patient is able to implement it. For example, a patient advised to swim to alleviate backache may be unable to swim, or the pool may be inaccessible or its entry fees unaffordable. Difficulties may also lie in the patient's belief in their 'Self Efficacy', their ability to enact the particular behaviour (Bandura 1977). With some forms of depression, the patient may have developed a crippling degree of learned helplessness. In our view, irrespective of the condition, doctors need to practise patient empowerment: reinforcing patients' ability to help themselves.

> Box 6.2   **As a result of your visit to the doctor today do you feel you are:**
>
> ◆ Able to cope with life?
> ◆ Able to understand your illness?
> ◆ Able to cope with your illness?
> ◆ Able to keep yourself healthy?
> ◆ Confident about your health?
> ◆ Able to help yourself?

Howie (Howie *et al.* 1997) has described the process of overcoming these barriers as 'Enablement' and has developed an instrument to measure this outcome (Box 6.2). It is not clear from his work what processes in the consultation enhance enablement, but other studies have provided clues. Encouragement, specific targets, reinforcing success, and shared decision making all contribute to a patient's belief in his or her own self-efficacy.

Task 5

To consider other problems:

(1) *not yet presented;*

(2) *continuing problems;*

(3) *at risk factors.*

This is quite clearly a more doctor-centred task and relates to the medical agenda. Patients may well not consult about all their problems, and may even not want them considered. Nevertheless, the doctor needs to think whether other problems may need to be raised. Continuity of care in general practice gives the doctor the opportunity to build up information about patients and their families that can be used to understand and contextualize the problems that have presented in subsequent consultations (Hjortdahl and Laerum 1992). In addition, there are many problems which patients continue to have, unrelated to the presenting problem, that the doctor may wish to raise. This is a complex decision and has to be handled both sensitively and with an eye to time. However well intentioned, insensitively raising continuing problems may obscure the immediate concern and prove to be counter productive.

Whatever the cause, many patients are at risk and the doctor has a role in disease prevention and health promotion. We agree with Nigel Stott and Robert Harvard Davies (1979) about 'opportunistic health promotion' and the exceptional potential of the primary care consultation. It is in this context that such matters can be raised as blood pressure checks, immunization status, and other screening activities. The opportunity to deliver preventive care to the population is one of the major strengths of primary care. The large majority of general practitioners have access to computers and these may make this task easier to achieve as prompts and reminders can be programmed and information readily accessed. On the other hand, the same group (Stott and Pill 1990) found that patients had reservations about doctor-driven health promotion, characterized by the response 'Advice yes, dictate no'.

Task 6

To use time appropriately:

(1) *in the consultation*;

(2) *in the longer term*.

Time is the general practitioner's principal resource, and it is usually rationed in 5, 10, or 15 min portions depending on the health care system. There is growing evidence that the length of the consultation is a major, but not the only, determinant, of its quality (Freeman *et al.* 2002). Ridsdale *et al.* (1992) showed that shorter consultations were less likely to contain any health promotion. Howie and colleagues (1999) showed that doctors who were able to enable their patients did so more effectively in longer consultations, while low enablers failed to increase their effectiveness with time. Thus, the issue of the appropriate use of time is fundamentally related to the other consultation tasks.

There are two issues: the length of the consultation and how well the available time is used. It is easy to believe that exploring the patients' agenda and perspective can be time consuming. It is also true that it may lead to economies in time as the consultation can then focus on the patient's needs. Many patients bring more than one item to the consultation, an increasing number bring a list. This can be used as a positive way of structuring and organizing the consultation to achieve the most effective use of time.

Little is known about the skilful use of time, but our experience has made it abundantly clear that some doctors can achieve the tasks effectively much quicker than others. Although this may seem to be obvious, the implications for training and monitoring are significant. We need to teach those strategies and skills that are most time efficient. For some it is a matter of practice but for others it seems that poor time management is caused by the clash of the doctor's and the patient's agendas. Clear consulting focus is a prerequisite of efficient time management.

Time is also a resource in the longer term and a major determinant of general practitioners workload is their return consultation rate. Patients who have had their problem explored fully, who understand it, and who are clear about how they can manage it themselves, are less likely to need to return. On the other hand 'safety netting' (ensuring that there is a clearly understood plan for when it is appropriate for the patient to return), is an essential part of good practice.

Task 7

To establish or maintain a relationship with the patient that helps to achieve the other tasks.

The essential point about this task is that it defines a desirable doctor–patient relationship in terms of its effectiveness rather than any preconceived ideas of correctness. According to this definition, an effective relationship is one in which the patient is able to state his or her ideas and concerns, in which sharing of information and decisions take place, and one in which a partnership between the patient and the doctor is built. As part of the evaluation of the patient enablement measure it was related to a measure of how well the patient knew the doctor. This relationship was highly predictive of the overall score: the longer the relationship on average, the better the score, though some good enablers were able to buck this trend (Howie *et al.* 1999). Kearley *et al.* (2001) also found that both patients and doctors valued a personal doctor–patient relationship, particularly for more serious or psychological problems.

A relationship can also be assessed in terms of its therapeutic effectiveness. As well as achieving the tasks, the extent to which a doctor displays warmth, genuineness, and unconditional regard for his patients also determines an effective therapeutic relationship (Rogers 1951; Novak 1987; Dixon *et al.* 1999).

There are also responsibilities on the doctor. Iona Heath in her book *Mystery of General Practice* (1995) identified three general responsibilities of the doctor, to interpret the patient's story, to act as the patient's guide at the interface of health and disease and to protect against over medicalization.

Roger Neighbour (1987) argues that doctors carry on an inner consultation in which there are two functions. The logical and rational part of the consulting activity is the domain of the organizer but the part that responds to the patient is different, more intuitive and more emotional. What happens to the relationship in the context of our tasks is that the doctor conducts an inner consultation, synthesizing the clinical evidence with the patient's narrative and constantly evaluating what needs to be said. This produces a dynamic, ever changing relationship, influenced by cognition, emotion, and feedback from the patient. This also means that relationships are influenced not only by what is said but how it is said.

The place of trust must also be crucial to outcome. Trust is not just perceived competence but also an evaluation of honesty and vested interest. Patients may distrust relationships which contain rationing implications and this may colour all the tasks. Per Fugelli (2001) stressed the importance of trust in the consultation and by implication the benefits of an ongoing partnership.

One of the biggest dangers to the doctor/patient relationship is the rise of defensive patterns in the consultation. Salinsky and Sackin have elucidated this area in their book '*What are you feeling doctor?*' (2000). They point out several defensive strategies used frequently by doctors to avoid emotional involvement. These include retreating totally into clinical medicine, always steering the conversation to the organic and so safely into tests, referrals, and prescriptions. Giving advice rather than listening, the deliberate use of protocols, policies, and the like, shield against the more difficult sharing of decisions.

There is also the danger of the relationship becoming too cosy, producing a state of dependency of one party on the other or even of mutual dependency. It may be that, to help doctors complete the tasks more effectively, they will need increased training in self-awareness, a greater recognition of the forces that create defensive patterns of consulting and greater help with emotional understanding. The tragedy that most vocational training (VT) remains remedial (Metcalfe 1999) is rooted in defensive and unhelpful patterns of consulting.

The effective relationship required to facilitate the tasks is not emotionally neutral. It carries emotional risk and requires real involvement with another human being: genuine enthusiasm and true caring.

Summary

In order to make the tasks more easily memorable, and more easily taught, we offer the following summary version of them:

- Understand the problem
- Understand the patient
- Share understanding
- Share decisions and responsibility
- Maintain the relationship

...and do all this within the allocated time!

7 Learning and teaching about the consultation

Introduction

In the previous chapter we have outlined the criteria for judging the effectiveness of a consultation. In this chapter we will consider how such an approach to consulting might best be taught and learned. We will first cover the theoretical principles upon which our approach is based, and then the ways that they can be applied to the consultation. The next two chapters will then describe the settings in which these approaches can be applied.

Theoretical principles

Learning

In our daily lives we frequently encounter new information, some of which challenges our established ways of understanding our world and ourselves. Whether we are children, adults, or professionals, we are well adapted to developing our understanding by incorporating new insights. This process requires effort to transform the new information into a form that is more easily assimilated into our existing mental schemes. When the new information does not fit easily within our existing knowledge, we have to reorganize our current understanding. Learning is a natural activity for us all, it may be easy or difficult, incidental or radical.

Children and adults learn in ways that are not identical but there are several important similarities. For example, people learn best when:

◆ they are motivated to learn
◆ what they need to learn is clear
◆ different learning methods or modalities are combined (e.g. by seeing, listening, talking, and doing), and the same coherent messages are drawn from each.

Kolb (1984) described how people learn.

(1) Experience: learning by involvement;
(2) Reflective: learning by review and thinking;

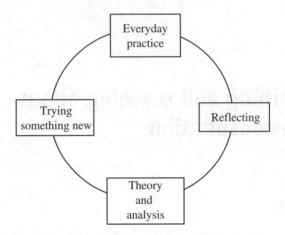

Fig. 7.1 Learning cycle.

(3)   Generalization: learning by reading and discussion;

(4)   Experiential or Testing: learning through activities.

People can learn in many different ways but by adulthood most people have demonstrated a preferred learning style. Nevertheless, learning involves several processes integrating activity with reflection, the discovery of new ideas, and experimentation to see how our performance might be improved. Figure 7.1 illustrates the point and is based on, but not identical to, Kolb's learning cycle.

Learning as adults and professionals

A number of factors can affect learning in adults when learning is meant to take place at the same time as professional practice (for a fuller discussion of these issues see Havelock *et al.* 1995):

1.   *Adults' concepts of themselves.* When adults see themselves essentially as having a function or task to perform, learning becomes a more peripheral activity

2.   *Self esteem.* Adults expect a certain status in society and in any group to which they belong. If the act of learning (or being in the 'learner' role) threatens that status, it is likely that learning opportunities will be bypassed

3.   *Previous experience.* When adult learners become busy and the pressures are on them, they are more likely to revert to previous behaviour rather than to think whether they should be proceeding differently and contemplating new ideas

4.   *Context and environment.* Learning will tend to happen more easily in an environment in which mutual learning and development is encouraged and nurtured: in which learning is the norm and is expected

5. *The learner's agenda.* Adults tend to take responsibility for what, how and when they learn. They normally only learn what they judge to be relevant and useful and at a time that seems appropriate.

The relationship between a teacher or tutor and someone who sees themselves as a learner is different from the relationship with someone who sees themselves as a fellow professional. Mezirow (1981) has provided guidelines for adult educators to help them structure their teaching so that this development in the relationship is encouraged.

1. *Progressively decrease the learner's dependency on the educator.* In this way learners become independent and more able to sustain their learning beyond the bounds of formal education.

2. *Help learners to use resources*—especially the experience of others—and to engage others in reciprocal learning relationships. In this way learning groups and teams are more likely to emerge.

3. *Assist learners to define their learning needs.* In this way learning becomes more self-directed and more efficient.

4. *Assist learners to assume increasing responsibility for defining their learning objectives, planning their own learning programme and evaluating their progress.* This is the final stage in the development of the self-directed learner.

We believe that these guidelines ensure that learners become self-directed and learning becomes self-sustaining throughout adult and professional life. Those responsible for managing and leading professional practice need to pay adequate attention to these matters in order to make learning more likely in the context of professional practice.

Developing competence

The principles we have outlined here fit well with the idea of continuing professional development. A profession may be variously defined but minimally it has a body of knowledge to which it lays claim, standards of skill and conduct that have to be maintained, and the capacity to regulate its own activities. Perhaps more importantly, a profession fosters a shared sense of purpose, shared values, and a duty of continuous learning.

Mature professionals, having once demonstrated their competence in their qualifying examinations, cannot presume to remain competent without continuing development. Yet professional development is frequently misunderstood. For many, it comprises updating of factual knowledge in the light of more recent advances in the evidence base. For us, professional development comprises the growth of experience and expertise. It might even be called the growth of wisdom.

As the professional observes practice, and reflects upon it, a number of further developments occur that are hard to teach formally. Taking a formal history, taught at medical school, becomes increasingly replaced by a more expert hypothetico-deductive method in which information is sought selectively to test the practitioner's hunches. Similarly, uncertainty is minimized by knowing when to deal with immediate problems and when to take the long view. Increasingly, account is taken of different contexts and of the background to the problem presented.

These processes seem not to be under conscious control for most professionals, yet they can be facilitated by colleagues. The difficulty is that expertise is frequently 'unconscious'. The growth of expertise has been described in four stages:

- unconscious incompetence
- conscious incompetence
- conscious competence
- unconscious competence.

Since expertise comprises unconscious competence, it is easily taken for granted. Continuous development frequently raises the level of consciousness, or awareness, in order to facilitate examination of, and reflection on, an aspect of performance. The learner feels awkward and the performance more laboured. In so doing, the level of demonstrated competence may also deteriorate temporarily, and the coach has to support the learner in order to encourage him/her not to retreat to the old ways and the old level of competence.

Figure 7.2 shows these principles schematically. It shows that the growth of expertise (or stable performance) is characteristically accompanied by a reduction in awareness. Once the coach intervenes to help improve performance, awareness

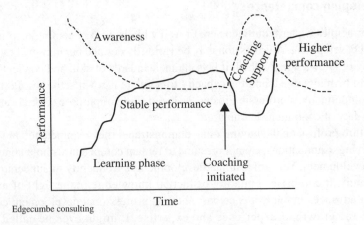

Edgecumbe consulting

Fig. 7.2 The relationship between awareness and performance.

instantly increases and performance may deteriorate until the new expertise has been assimilated and the level of awareness has once again dropped to low levels. All sportsmen and sportswomen know this experience intimately.

Our approach to learning and teaching

We have drawn from the foregoing brief résumé of educational ideas a few key principles upon which our own approach has been based:

1. Make teaching learner centred

The aims of our teaching are to help doctors to be able to conduct more effective consultations, and to be able to continue to maintain and improve their effectiveness in the future. We have defined effectiveness as being able to achieve the tasks described in Chapter 6, and the first step in any teaching is to share this model as a clear statement of what is to be learned.

When the definition of effective consulting has been agreed, the task of the teacher is to help a specific learner to raise his or her game. This implies that the baseline of the individual's current level of performance is the point of departure for the learning and teaching process. Each individual's baseline is unique and needs to be assessed early in the relationship between teacher and learner.

The learner's agenda is also important, but it is not overriding. We also believe in the teacher's expertise. The teacher has to respond to the learner's agenda but not be dominated by it, helping the learner understand what needs to be learned. The teacher thus needs to teach *through* the learner's agenda helping to expand, question, and fashion that agenda, rather than either ignoring it or following it blindly.

2. Choose methods appropriate for the message

Messages can be reinforced when teachers use a variety of different teaching methods to facilitate learning. Patient involvement in decision-making may be approached in a tutorial or through reading to develop a theoretical base, in a small group session to discuss attitudes and feelings, and by using video-feedback to develop skills. The skilful teacher selects the medium that best carries a coherent message and employs other compatible methods for reinforcement rather than attempting to use a favourite method to fit all lessons.

3. Preach what you practise

Learner centred teaching reinforces patient-centred consulting. Shared decision-making in the consultation needs to be modelled in the teacher–learner relationship. Modelling fosters learning whether or not it is intended and the burden on the teacher is to demonstrate in everyday practice the lessons he/she wishes to be learned. In this way, the learner experiences the thoughts and feelings needed to apply the learning. The principle of preaching what you practise (a more difficult challenge than practising what you preach) emphasises the responsibility of the teacher to seek always to put his or her house in order first. Certainly, 'do as I say, not as I do' is ineffective.

4. Integrate learning and practice

Learning must be based on previous experience and the needs identified in practice, and must provide the opportunities for change in future practice. These links may need to be made explicitly. Opportunities for experimentation and practice need to be created, and permission to risk disruption of established practice, and even initial failure, needs to be given.

5. Establish a learning culture

Continuous learning comprises intellectual curiosity, enthusiasm for improvement, and a mind that remains open to new possibilities. It also requires willingness to try something new. These principles are best learned as early in professional life as possible. They are the learning habits that will last for a professional lifetime.

The teacher needs to develop a culture in the work place that enables learning. Mistakes can be made into learning opportunities or they can provoke blame and guilt. Time for teaching can be protected or it can be seen as a soft activity that can readily be interrupted or postponed. Professional colleagues can give the impression that they welcome feedback and want to raise their game continuously, or that they are 'fully fledged' and now above improvement or scrutiny. A learning culture makes development the norm.

Applying these principles to learning about the consultation

The stages involved in applying these principles in practice can be summarized as follows:

1. Engage and involve the learner. Engage the learners, establish their agenda and agree to proceed.

2. *Present a rationale for the tasks.* Present a rationale for the consultation tasks, and negotiate their acceptability related to the learner's own experience of practice.

3. *Observe and describe the consultation.* Describe the content of the consultation and recognize when a particular task is being attempted.

4. *Evaluate.* Assess the extent to which each task was achieved in a consultation.

5. *Provide constructive feedback.* Identify how the tasks were achieved and the reasons why any task was not being fully achieved, and consider how this can be improved.

6. *Develop self-awareness.* Help the learner evaluate their own effectiveness, and to identify the thoughts and feelings that they have during the consultation.

7. *Choose appropriate learning strategies.* Agree future learning needs and the most appropriate methods of meeting them.

8. *Experiment and practice.* Encourage the learner to practice the proposed changes both in protected settings and with their patients.

We will now consider each of these stages in turn.

Engage the learner

We now know that, in order for communication teaching to work, we really must begin with the learner. Whether in big groups, small groups, or individuals it is necessary to engage with the audience. We tell consulting anecdotes and encourage the learners to recall their experiences. We can admit to an element of evangelism in our enthusiasm for patient-centred medicine and consider that pursuing the religious metaphor may be helpful in understanding the teaching and learning process. We have found that the majority of our audiences pay lip service to the values and concepts of task based, patient-centred medicine, but as we have pointed out elsewhere, the performance often seems to lag far behind.

True patient-centred medicine depends on a significant shift in attitudes and thinking. This conversion may not happen before taking the academic and practical steps to modify the learner's consulting but is far more likely to occur if the learner has a good learning experience.

It can help a session to begin with the audience. A question such as 'What kind of consultations do you find hard?' or 'What does patient-centred medicine mean to you?' will stimulate a lively discussion. In a lecture theatre, the audience can quickly be divided into trios and each individual given an allotted time of say 5 min. This breaks the ice, turns a lecture into a participative experience and provides much material for the subsequent talk. We have found that humour is a great facilitator and enlivens as it lightens the learning.

Presenting and agreeing the tasks

Our tasks define an effective consultation. Teaching begins by helping the learner understand the tasks and both their theoretical background and their evidence base. This discussion may lead to disagreement about the tasks. Patients' involvement in decision-making may seem inappropriate, achieving the tasks within the timeframe of usual general practice may seem impossible. These issues need to be worked through and resolved, both theoretically and practically, so that the task list becomes a *shared* definition of an effective consultation. We have found that a number of different methods may be required at this early stage to reach a shared agreement to use the tasks as criteria for the consultation. For example, it might need:

◆ further reading of the evidence

◆ experimentation with the method to test its feasibility

◆ a discussion about values and attitudes supported by other literature

◆ a different approach to practice management (e.g. slightly longer appointments or no interruptions during the consultations).

More often than not, the most important breakthrough comes from seeing the tasks in action: from a demonstration.

Observing and describing a consultation

Description is fundamentally different from evaluation. When we describe a consultation we merely attempt to produce a record of events that are taking place. When we evaluate the same consultation we attempt to judge how effectively important matters were handled.

In order to become familiar with the seven consultation tasks, we have devised the technique of *consultation mapping*. This approach was first described in our earlier volume. Mapping is a technique for describing the progress of a consultation through the tasks. It is possible to describe other matters in a consultation. For example, we may describe the non-verbal behaviour or the feelings in a consultation but these descriptions, although valid, are not yet pertinent to our purposes. Subsequently we shall want to know *why* the consultation was as it was but, for the moment, we simply want to learn to recognize attempts to achieve each task in order that we may subsequently evaluate it.

Each time the doctor or the patient speaks, what is said may be placed under the heading of one of our tasks (unless it is totally irrelevant). Consider the following extract from a consultation:

> *Patient*: Well doctor, I've been having trouble with my ears. They're really painful. Well, the right one's painful, the other one's OK now.
> *Doctor*: How long has that been going on?
> *Patient*: About a week now.
> *Doctor*: Have you noticed anything else?
> *Patient*: Well, I've had a bit of soreness in my throat.
> *Doctor*: What do you think has given you the earache?
> *Patient*: I've been swimming a lot lately and I wondered if I might have got a bit of an infection.
> *Doctor*: Let me have a look in your ears.

In this brief extract, the patient begins by offering information about the nature and history of the problem. The doctor's first two questions and the patient's answers follow up this matter. When the doctor asks what the patient thinks may have caused the earache, he is beginning to explore the patient's ideas and when

Task 1. To understand the reasons for the patient's attendance, including the patient's problem and the patient's perspective	
a. The patient's problem: nature and history	O———o———o———o o——
aetiology	
effects	
b. The patient's perspective: personal and social circumstances	
ideas and values about health	
ideas about the problem, it's causes and its management	
concerns about the problem and it's implications	
expectations for information, involvement, and care.	

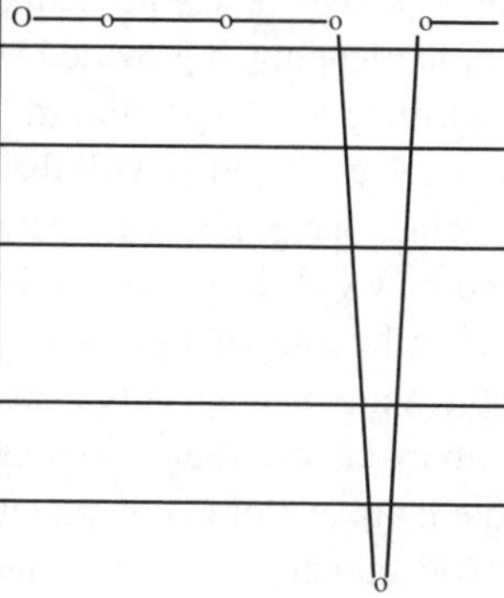

Fig. 7.3 Mapping the consultation.

he examines the ears, he is retuning to the nature and history of the problem. This extract might be plotted as on the attached map of the consultation (Fig 7.3).

Here we can immediately see some of the difficulties in categorization. When the doctor asked 'What do you think has given you the earache?' was he seeking ideas from the patient or was he considering the aetiology of the problem? Clearly, this matter needs to be resolved by asking the doctor but while the consultation is in progress we need to make the best guess we can. The map is not a precise tool, but it will leave a reasonable record of the sequence of events. If the learner and teacher complete a map of the same consultation the differences can highlight different perceptions and form the basis for significant discussion and learning.

Similarly, more than one thing may be happening at any given time. For example, as the doctor is systematically exploring the nature and history of a problem, the patient's understanding of it may be increasing. Thus, the observer may wish to make an entry in more than one category in response to just one brief portion of the consultation. If the consultation is recorded on videotape, such matters may be resolved as and when they arise and, as a teacher and a learner get to know each other, such problems usually arise less often. Other problems might also need to be resolved such as whether to record questions as well as answers or whether to record the intention of a question or the answer given which may not have been intended. The point is that there is not a preferable way of mapping a consultation, merely an agreed way.

In order to map a consultation, we take all of the tasks except numbers 6 and 7 (to use time appropriately and to establish or maintain a helpful relationship) and set out each part separately. We exclude the sixth and seventh tasks since they cannot be seen at any particular time in the consultation. The form used for consultation mapping is provided below.

By describing a consultation in this way we become more familiar with the tasks themselves and also with the doctor's attempts to achieve them. There is no clear relationship, however, between how often a doctor attempts to achieve a task and how well it is done. A doctor may ask ten questions about the effects of a problem but may not put any of them clearly with the result that the effects of a problem are inadequately explored. Another doctor may ask just two questions but may choose them so carefully and put them so well that the effects of the problem are explored completely.

When the learner is new to the tasks, and to the mapping exercise, we recommend using the tasks in summary format. In this case, the mapping form is shown in Box 7.1.

Naturally, lessons using this format are few and easily learned but we would expect that this format would prompt the teacher and learner to resolve how they intend to mark the map and also to see how rarely most inexperienced doctors share decision-making with patients.

After one or two consultations have been mapped in this way, the learner and teacher will want to progress to the full map, which looks like Box 7.2.

Many consultations, especially in General Practice, contain multiple problem presentations. To distinguish these on the same map, other symbols, or different coloured pencils can be used. If the videotape does not have a time stamp, it is easy to annotate the video recorder index numbers at points on the map of significant interest to allow easy replay. After completion of the consultation, all the crosses and other symbols can be joined together sequentially using a ruler. With a little practice, it is possible to map consultations of colleagues while

---

Box 7.1 **Short consultation map**

Each time the doctor or the patient speaks, place a mark against the appropriate heading. These marks may then be joined together so that the sequence of events in the consultation is made clear.

Understand the patient's problem
Understand the patient's perspective
Share understanding about the problem
  and the options for management
Share decision making about management
Involve the patient

Box 7.2   **Complete consultation map**

Each time the doctor or the patient speaks, place a mark against the appropriate heading. These marks may then be joined together so that the sequence of events in the consultation is made clear.

Task 1. To understand the reasons for the patient's attendance, including the patient's problem and the patient's perspective:
a. The patient's problem:
   Nature and history
   Aetiology
   Effects
b. The patient's perspective:
   Personal and social
     circumstances
   Ideas and values about
     health
   Ideas about the problem,
     it's causes and its
     management
   Concerns about the
     problem and it's
     implications
   Expectations for
     information,
     involvement, and care

Task 2. Taking into account the patient's perspective, to achieve a shared understanding:
About the problem
About the evidence and
  options for management

Task 3. To enable the patient to choose an appropriate action for each problem:
Consider options and
  implications
Choose the most
  appropriate course of action

Task 4: To enable the patient to manage the problem:
Discuss the patient's ability
  to take appropriate actions
Agree doctor and patient
  actions and responsibilities
Agree targets, monitoring
  and follow up

Task 5. To consider other problems:
Not yet presented
Continuing problems
At risk factors

their consultations are in progress. This gives a permanent record without technology and stops a lot of arguments about what did and did not occur.

The completed consultation map should be used in a similar way to a road map; it will describe the behaviours visited and the ones which were not, but it will not by itself describe the quality or effectiveness of those behaviours. Road maps do not say whether it was a pretty village or an ugly, run-down place: the observer has to make that quality judgement. Just so with the consultation map. A map may show a 10-min examination, but it is up to the observers to judge how appropriate and effective that examination was. The map only shows that the behaviour was present or absent. This method has been used in more formal attempts to assess the content and quality of consultations (Hays 1990; Arborelius and Bremberg 1992).

After the mapping exercise has been completed, one might legitimately want to judge how well each task was achieved. We shall deal with this in the next section. However, because of its sequential nature, a series of maps of an individual consulting can be very revealing. Several maps demonstrate the doctor's style in action and demonstrates regularities. The doctor may say: 'Oh yes, patients' concerns are important, I was a bit rushed this time, but I will definitely ask him next time'. The series of maps may reveal that tomorrow never comes.

Used in this way the map is a guide to performance by demonstrating, quite unequivocally, the tasks that are attempted and those that are not. To us, the most worrying common pattern in young registrars is a recurrent absence of an entry in the personal and social circumstances line. We are family doctors and pride ourselves on our knowledge of our patients and their families. To achieve this knowledge over time we have to seek out personal information, so that each consultation becomes a brick in a wall. If there are no bricks there can be no wall. The map will identify pivotal moments in the interchange, which can then be analysed at leisure. The map can be improved by writing notes or prompts on it at the appropriate places; snippets of conversation, significant words used, what the problems were such as 'sore throat, goitre, unhappy, etc.'

A method for evaluating a consultation

In order to evaluate a consultation, we have devised a *consultation rating scale*. This is based on the consultation tasks in the same way, as is the consultation map. It is essential to complete the map first. Our experience has shown us that behaviours that were in fact absent in the consultation can still be zealously rated by some inexperienced learners. Each individual part of each task is rated separately and we have chosen to set our the rating scale in the form of opposing statements linked by a line. The rater is asked to place a mark (/) on the line in such a way that it represents how much he agrees with the opposing statements. The first pair of statements is:

Nature and history of (a)   (b)   (c)   Nature and history
problems adequately .../...................... of problems defined
defined   inadequately.

If the rater thought that the nature and history of the problems had been defined adequately, he might place his mark at point (a). If he thought that the nature and history had been inadequately defined, he might place his mark at (c). If he thought that the nature and history of the problem had been defined in part but that more should have been established in order for the nature and history to have been adequate he might place his mark at point (b). In most general practice consultations, however, more than one problem is presented. In this case, instead of placing a mark on the scale, the rater might want to place a 1 when he is rating the way in which the first problem was dealt with, a 2 when rating the way in which the second problem was handled and so on.

This kind of scale has the advantage that a wide range of opinions may be expressed. Small differences may also be recorded although this is only an advantage if the judgements are reliably made. It has the disadvantage that a judge can always use the midpoint and never commit himself to a firm opinion but this disadvantage is removed when recommendations have to be made. We shall describe this more fully in the following section on feedback. The consultation rating scale is provided in Box 7.3.

It is important to understand how the words 'adequately' and 'appropriately' have been used in the rating scale. Here they are seen more often than in the original list of tasks. If we take that part of the scale, which deals with the exploration of the effects of the problem(s), we may first want to judge whether the effects of the problems should have been explored at all. If the effects of a problem cause particular distress, such as the disruption of a happy home, and if these effects have recently been explored at great length, it may be inappropriate to explore them in the present consultation. In these circumstances, a skilled exploration of the effects of the problem may be marked down on the grounds of inappropriateness. More commonly, if an exploration of the effects of a problem was entirely appropriate but not carried out adequately, the rater will mark down this aspect of the consultation on the grounds of inadequacy. Thus, *either* an inappropriate *or* an inadequate exploration will be marked down.

Giving feedback

Much has been made of the rules for feedback dubbed the Pendleton rules. The key to effective feedback is to offer both challenge and support but the rules are often used as reasons to be supportive without being challenging. Here, we want to explore how to provide feedback that preserves self-esteem but which

Box 7.3 **Complete consultation rating scale**

After the consultation has ended, please rate the achievement of the tasks by placing a mark on each scale provided.

Task 1. To understand the reasons for the patient's attendance, including the patient's problem and the patient's perspective:
a. The patient's problem:

Nature and history defined adequately	Nature and history defined inadequately
Aetiology defined adequately	Aetiology defined inadequately
effects defined adequately	Effects defined inadequately

b. The patient's perspective:

Personal and social circumstances defined adequately	Personal and social circumstances defined inadequately
Ideas and values about health defined adequately	Ideas and values about health defined inadequately
Ideas about the problem, it's causes and its management defined adequately	Ideas about the problem, it's causes and its management defined inadequately
Concerns about the problem and it's implications defined adequately	Concerns about the problem and it's implications defined inadequately
Expectations for information, involvement, and care defined adequately	Expectations for information, involvement, and care defined inadequately

Task 2. Taking into account the patient's perspective, to achieve a shared understanding:

Shared understanding about the problem achieved adequately and appropriately	Shared understanding about the problem achieved inadequately or inappropriately
Shared understanding about the evidence and options for management achieved adequately and appropriately	Shared understanding about the evidence and options for management achieved inadequately or inappropriately

Task 3. To enable the patient to choose an appropriate action for each problem:

Options and implications considered adequately and appropriately	Options and implications considered inadequately or inappropriately
The most appropriate course of action chosen adequately and appropriately	The most appropriate course of action chosen inadequately or inappropriately

Task 4: To enable the patient to manage the problem:

Patient's ability to take appropriate actions discussed adequately	Patient's ability to take appropriate actions discussed inadequately

| Doctor and patient agreed actions and responsibilities adequately | Doctor and patient agreed actions and responsibilities inadequately |
| Targets, monitoring and follow up agreed adequately | Targets, monitoring and follow up agreed inadequately |

Task 5. To consider other problems:

Problems not yet presented considered adequately	Problems not yet presented considered inadequately
Continuing problems considered adequately	Continuing problems considered inadequately
At risk factors considered adequately	At risk factors considered inadequately

also challenges the learner to develop, improve, and grow. The process seeks to understand how and why certain tasks are done well and others are not.

The rules we first published in our 1984 book suggested that feedback should:

(1)   Briefly clarify any matters of fact (but no rhetorical questions please!)

(2)   Encourage the learner to go first

(3)   Consider what has been done well first

(4)   Make recommendations rather than state weaknesses.

These were drafted almost as an afterthought when the book was first published. They were devised as a corrective to the erstwhile medical school norm of teaching through humiliation. They implied that learners need to be in control of their learning to a significant extent, that building on strengths is more effective than focusing on weaknesses, and that suggestions are easier to assimilate than are lists of stated weaknesses.

Above all, the rules were designed to create a safe environment in which learners could respond more positively to recommendations, avoiding defensiveness. This would be an environment in which learners could take risks in their development and experiment without fear. Yet several accounts of the way the rules are used give rise to concern. Two in particular stand out. The first when the rules are used without explicit criteria and the second when they are used as laws rather than guidelines.

When the rules are used without explicit criteria, they are incomplete. When a consultation needs to be evaluated, our intention is that the seven tasks be used as evaluation criteria as described above. Merely to ask what went well, without the tasks as a yardstick, leaves the criteria unclear, and the learner vulnerable to unexpected criticism—an ambush.

When the rules are used as laws rather than guidelines, they are inappropriately dogmatized. Silverman and colleagues (Kurtz *et al.* 1998) have suggested that the rules artificially constrain the feedback so that the learning suffers. Their criticism centres on the 'strict ordering of feedback' that 'creates an artificiality about the feedback process' and that the rules 'seem to suggest that ensuring safety through the strict observance of the order of contribution is of more importance than enabling an interactive discussion' (p. 291). Not surprisingly, they are also critical of the implied criticism of making recommendations, the postponement of discovering the learner's agenda and the inefficient use of time working in this way.

The guidelines we proposed are best seen as principles rather than laws. Most of the points made by Silverman *et al.* reflect over-zealous application of the feedback principles originally suggested. Discovering the learner's agenda really helps and this should happen early in the learning process. We call this process 'contracting' but we did not write about it in the first edition. A contract needs to be agreed at the start of any feedback process, or any teaching session. The contract covers:

- the timeframe for the discussion
- the learner's agenda
- the teacher's agenda
- roles and responsibilities.

We firmly believe in the learner-centred approach and we believe it is more effective to build on strengths. Thus it makes sense to establish the strengths (good points) of the consultation first. This works well as a collaborative exercise when the feedback is taking place in a group setting. The aim here is not mere politeness or uncritical acclaim. *The aim is to understand how and why certain consultation tasks were achieved.* Understanding how these successes were brought about enables the same ends to be achieved at will on

Box 7.4	**Positive and negative feedbacks**		
		Positive feedback (preserves or enhances the learner's self respect)	Negative feedback (reduces the learner's self respect)
	Feedback about good performance	✓	X
	Feedback about performance that needs to be (or could be) improved	✓	X

future occasions. This brings the process more under control and builds a real skill base.

Positive feedback is to be distinguished from uncritical feedback. *Positive feedback preserves or enhances the learner's self respect*, thus freeing them up to the possibility of change and improvement without harm. Negative feedback threatens the learner's self respect and creates defensive resistance. It inhibits learning and is counter-productive.

Feedback needs to comment both on good performance and on those aspects that could or should be improved. It needs to be direct and positive at all times. The point is best made in Box 7.4.

Positive feedback about good performance looks like this:

> When you explained that the stomach pain could not have been caused by indigestion, you incorporated her ideas and used her own words effectively. You made a real contribution to her understanding of her health.
>
> The patient seemed to be at ease with you and she did not seem at all embarrassed explaining her concerns at some length.

Positive feedback about performance that needs to be improved looks like this:

> Instead of explaining so much all at once, I think it would have been better to cover only the first two points you made.
>
> I think you may have needed to find out more about her ideas. You may have asked her to tell you how she thought the pain began. This would have let you go on to explore her concerns more fully.

By contrast, negative feedback feels very different. For example, negative feedback about good performance looks like this:

> You normally overcomplicate your explanations. This time you didn't do that. Why can't you always explain like this, so your patients stand a chance of remembering some of what you told them?
>
> Once you started to concentrate and get yourself organised, the consultation went quite well.

Negative feedback about performance that needs to be improved looks like this:

> If I've told you once, I've told you a thousand times, don't just tell your patients what to do—discuss the options and make a choice together. You didn't do that here and you don't usually.
>
> Are you sure you're really cut out for general practice?

The purpose of feedback is well summarized by Jenny King (1999) in these terms: 'Giving feedback is not just to provide a judgement or evaluation. It is to provide insight. Without insight into their own strengths and limitations (trainees) cannot progress or resolve difficulties' (p. 2). She also outlined the criteria for judging feedback to be effective. She suggested that feedback should be:

(1) *Descriptive* of the behaviour rather than the personality;

(2) *Specific* rather than general;

(3) *Sensitive* to the needs of the receiver as well as the giver;

(4) *Directed* towards behaviour that can be changed;

(5) *Timely*: given as close to the event as possible while taking into account the learner's readiness; and

(6) *Selective*: addressing one or two key issues rather than too many at once.

We recommend that feedback principles are treated as such, rather than elevated to the status of dogma. The one principle that needs to come above all others, however, is that learning is easier when self-esteem is preserved or enhanced and when success and failure are both adequately understood. We advocate directness and sensitivity.

Developing self awareness

Giving feedback in this way will help the learner become more aware of their own strengths and areas that need improvement. Effective consulting is not however just a collection of behaviours, it is also a relationship between two people in which thoughts and feelings direct events. A number of specific approaches have been developed to help doctors become more aware, and therefore more able to interpret and control, those feelings.

Inter-personal process recall (IPPR)

This is a specific training technique developed by Norman Kagan (1969) in which the role of the teacher is as an *enquirer* inviting the doctor to recall what they were thinking or feeling at each stage in a recorded interview. The doctor identifies the significant points in the interview and the enquirer is there to promote reflection and not to teach behaviours. The aim is to develop the doctor's self-awareness and to establish greater control over their feelings.

A Consultation self-appraisal proforma

This has been developed by Roger Neighbour (Personal communication) as a method of describing the events of the consultation. It has to be completed afterwards and can only be completed by the participant. Again the map can be used to jog the memory and give the time scale, but it is better if the consultation has been audio or video recorded and it can be reviewed slowly, stopping frequently. The learner reviews the recording (or MAP) of the consultation and stops the tape after each minute of elapsed time, and then describes what happens in each successive minute. The idea of this device is to highlight the learner's own perceptions of what occurred, and why. This tool, unlike the map, also lends itself to exploring the developing relationship between the doctor and the patient. The following example (Box 7.5) is a male patient of 58 who the doctor did not know very well, but whose elderly mother he saw regularly. This was the last appointment on a busy Friday evening.

Box 7.5	**Consultation self-appraisal proforma**
Time in minutes	Observations
0–1	I am tense and one hour late. He wants tablets to calm the blood down! I think he is anxious and need to hear more. I let him talk.
1–2	He tells me of his moles. I ask a couple of questions seeking the cause of his irritation. I think he is very afraid of cancer.
2–3	He tells me more about his moles & I examine him, both a clinical and a therapeutic procedure. I tell him moles are not irritating.
3–4	I carry on examining him get a bit more history and now he tells me about his friend who died of a cancerous mole.
4–5	I check his medication in search for cause of the irritation, temazepam rears its ugly head. We both note it and pass on.
5–6	I pause, tap the desk, consciously stopping in order to clarify and review where we have got to. I involve him in the management decision.
6–7	I suggest, long windedly, that in view of the worry I will take off his moles.
7–8	He talks about his friend, he is quite frightened.
8–9	He asks me how can I tell the difference between a bad mole and a good one. I embark on an explanation.
9–10	I'm still explaining. It is rather one sided. I do not check his understanding and ignore some verbal clues.
10–11	He tells me for the last year he has been frightened to strip off in the sun. I say make appointment for minor op and histology will confirm all OK.
11–12	He wants to talk about his frail mother. I am tired, reluctant to say too much but share some of my thoughts.
12–13	He is kind to me and I feel uneasy. He lets me know that he is worried about mother but appreciates there is no medical easy answer.
13–14	He leaves and I wish I had been quicker about his moles and longer about his mother.

This is essentially a descriptive tool, but it forces doctors to collect their thoughts about the events. It may be the best tool for unearthing values and beliefs, and with a skilled teacher all sorts of sensitive topics can be raised and discussed. The map, rating scale, critique, and this proforma are complimentary.

Other methods have been found to be effective in developing the doctors' personal attributes. Attitudes can be modified by peer group discussion, and an extended period of structured discussion of cases focussing on the doctor's reactions to the patient's problems can lead to 'A modified change in personality' (Balint 1957).

Teaching strategies

There may be many reasons why someone is unable to carry out an effective consultation, as discussed in Chapter 5, *Understanding the Doctor*:

1. It might be that he/she does not understand or have *knowledge* of what is needed to be done; for example—a doctor that does not know that anger is part of a normal bereavement reaction and thus reacts inappropriately to a patient's outburst.

2. It might be that the doctor's *values or beliefs* make them resistant to exploring something that is of importance to a patient; for example—a doctor who believes that depression is a 'chemical disorder of the brain' and does not discuss possible causative factors for low mood in a patient.

3. It might be that a doctor does not have the range of *strategies or skills* to deal with the patients presenting symptom; for example—when confronted with a patient with symptoms of anxiety, the doctor can only prescribe because he has not acquired the range of other managements such as cognitive approaches or counselling. Similarly, the doctor might not be able to use open questions and silence in consultations

4. It might be that a doctor has other *distractors* that are affecting the effectiveness of the consultation either general or patient related; for example— the doctor who is stressed by the organization of the surgery or by domestic issues might reject cues offered by the patients and be unable to concentrate fully on the issues presented.

5. It might be that a doctor has had *negative feedback* from, or difficulties with, a certain group of patients and feels dissatisfied with other similar patients; for example—a doctor has had a number of unsatisfactory consultations with women concerning their menopause and therefore is likely to consult badly with patients with menopausal symptoms.

These examples show the importance of the diagnostic approach to teaching effective consultations. Each of them would require different teaching methods and approaches. There is a very high level of skill in an effective doctor/patient consultation, something that is often minimized by those trying to analyse or teach consultations.

Learners usually need help to find ways of developing their consultations, whether through a discussion about the ethics of the issues raised, or through the development of a specific skill. Over time, the learning needs of a doctor will change and their agenda will also develop. An effective teacher needs to change method and content of teaching to match these learner needs, using different types of consultations as the need arises.

Opportunities for practice

Previously we have possibly under-emphasized the need for practice. Now is the time to redress that balance. Consulting well is a complex skill, like playing a musical instrument. No one wakes up in the morning suddenly being able to play the piano; it requires tuition and repetitive practice. We believe good consulting is no different.

Simulated patients or role plays, even with the teacher, can provide the opportunity for the learner to rehearse a new skill rather than just talk about it. This allows the learner to see whether a new approach actually works for them, and reinforces the learning.

Introducing a new behaviour into real consultations can be difficult and may fail at the first attempt. For example if it is agreed that the learner would like to explore the patient's ideas about their problem the first attempt may be to ask 'What do you think is wrong with you?' with the predictable response 'You tell me, you are the doctor'. More skilful questions need to be rehearsed beforehand, 'What thoughts have been going through your mind?'. The learner needs encouragement to try more than once and to identify the positive reinforcement that patients can give. In this way 'conscious competence' will be developed.

Observing consultations

So far we have talked about observing consultations without considering which consultations they should be. In our first (1984) volume, we included a chapter wholly devoted to observing the consultation and the mechanisms of effective production of a videotape of 'real' consultations. Technology has moved on since then, equipment has developed from the original analogue reel-to-reel tape recorders to digital and beyond, the acceptance by doctors and patients of the technique is established and videotapes are widely used in educational and professional examinations. Methods for gaining informed consent have been debated and agreed. Appropriate technical quality of a video recording can now easily be achieved and the standards are widely accepted. It would be inappropriate for this book to go further into these subjects except to emphasize their importance in order to facilitate effective learning and teaching.

Use of role-play and actors

In addition to observing real consultations, either directly or on video, we have found the use of role play and actors to be an important part of a consultation teacher's repertoire. We have also noticed that there has been a great increase in the use of actors, role players, and simulated patients since 1984. A good role player can bring to the teaching session the feelings, frustrations and joys that a patient might experience. They also enable the learner to re-do part or all of the consultation after the feedback and this enables the practice and development of new skills.

Role players also bring a patient perspective. Those who do it on a regular basis bring a view that has been accumulated from many consultations with different types of health care workers about a wide range of issues. They can share with the learner the feelings, frustrations, and joys that a patient might experience in the protected environment of the teaching session. Another strength of role playing from a known script is the identification of the patient's agenda. In actual consultations this is always a matter for conjecture and debate, often leading to fruitless discussions of what the patient's 'real' agenda was. In role playing the true agenda is known and level of task completion can be unequivocally identified. This makes it a very powerful methodology for demonstrating consulting behaviours.

Summary

Essential to learning to consult effectively are: criteria for an effective consultation, a means of observing real performance and positive feedback about those tasks that have been achieved, and those that need to be improved. Establishing a learning culture in the practice accelerates the learning and the most powerful learning comes from observing skilful practice.

8 Putting the tasks into practice

Introduction

One of the most crucial issues we face is the gap between the rhetoric advocating patient centred consulting and the clear evidence that this is still not widespread in practice. Successive studies in British general practice have painted a consistent and relatively unchanging picture of consultations lasting between 5 and 10 min in which patients' ideas are not explored, explanations and choices are not offered, and decisions are not shared (Byrne and Long 1964; Tuckett *et al*. 1985; Makoul *et al*. 1995; Stevenson *et al*. 2000). In Chapter 5 we have described some of the factors that influence how doctors consult, including their own beliefs and skills, the environment in which the consultation takes place, as well as the consultation itself and its outcome. All of these may be considered as potential levers for change.

In this chapter we will examine these issues from the point of view of the individual doctor in practice. This chapter will help those doctors who look at the tasks laid out in Chapter 6 and feel that they are either impossible or difficult to incorporate into their daily consultations. We will draw on the experience of working with many thousands of doctors over the years and describe the techniques that have been found useful. It is difficult to change long established consulting habits. The 'Readiness to Change' model described by Prochaska and DiClemente (1983) has been the basis of many approaches to changing patients' behaviour. However, this approach is rarely applied to doctors, who are usually exhorted to change, and blamed when they fail to do so.

Here, we will consider the stages the individual doctor would need to go through to make changes in the way that he or she consults with patients, including coping with the stresses that change produces. We will also consider how the environment within which the doctor works can be developed to support a patient-centred approach.

Readiness to change

The Readiness to Change Model (Box 8.1) includes a number of stages and each is dependent on the previous stage. It starts with a *Pre-contemplation* stage: when change has not been considered and the status quo is completely acceptable.

Box 8.1   **The Readiness to change model**

- Pre-contemplation
- Contemplation
- Preparation
- Action
- Maintenance

Contemplation is the start of awareness of the need to change. During the *Preparation* stage, the will to change emerges as the pros outweigh the cons. It is the stage in which plans are made. *Action* describes the process of change with all its attendant difficulties. The final stage, *Maintenance*, includes the process of incorporating the change into daily life and ensuring that it is sustained.

Pre-contemplation: everything is ok

There are many doctors in Britain who are unaware of the benefits of patient-centred consulting for their patients and themselves. It might not be a subject that they have considered, or they may have considered it and think that they are practising patient-centred consulting effectively. It could be that the pressures of their lives and the difficulties of practice do not allow them the contemplation space to consider their consultations. They are too busy *doing*, to reflect on the process. Many of the factors that keep a doctor in the pre-contemplation phase are considered in Chapter 5.

Contemplation: why change?

The first stage in changing is to become aware of the need for change. We know that the least effective way to get patients to stop smoking or lose weight is to tell them to do so repeatedly. People are persuaded in different ways. Some people are convinced by published evidence. Doctors who are persuaded by this kind of evidence may find the literature reviewed in earlier chapters in this book to be persuasive. Most people need to accept that change is important to them, and that the rewards outweigh the costs. They also need to be confident that they can do what is required. We are all too keenly aware that persuasion without enablement will ultimately be frustrating.

A doctor who just likes to try things and who trusts his/her own experience may want to try out some of the aspects of patient-centred consulting we have described earlier. Such a doctor may experiment by asking a few patients about their thoughts and their concerns, or by asking them for their opinion about possible treatment options. In many cases, just the exploration of the patient's story about her condition will give new insights into the person and provide clues about how to consult more effectively.

Many doctors still regard consultation as an art. They believe that this art is an innate gift, or that it has developed over years with experience. This view tends to be an obstacle to change. The change to patient-centred consulting involves a shift of power from the doctor to the patient and this can make some doctors feel uncomfortable or even threatened. In this case it is easier to see patients as 'patients' and not as people with lives outside the consulting room.

Byrne and Long's early work analysing consultations concentrated on style and coined the phrases doctor-centred and patient-centred (Byrne and Long 1976). They concluded that doctors were quite fixed in their style and that how they consulted was unrelated to either the type of patient or the condition presented. The differences in style were personal to the doctor. One doctor might be able to listen well and encourage a patient to talk while another might be able to explain effectively and increase the patient's understanding. Nevertheless, the predominant style was doctor-centred.

Developing skills in consultations allows the doctor to develop a range of styles to tailor consultations more to the patient and the presenting condition. These are matters of behaviour, not personality. Personality is relatively fixed, but skills can be learned. Some people might naturally have a personality that makes effective listening more difficult, but everyone can improve their skills. Byrne and Long described the doctor's style as 'a prison in which a doctor works'. Broadening the range of consulting skills allows the doctor to escape from that prison to the benefit of doctor and patients alike.

Planning: what changes do I want to make?

Wanting to change to a patient-centred style of consulting is not enough; we need to develop the appropriate skills. These are not entirely new skills specifically developed for patient-centred consultations, they are largely interpersonal skills learned since childhood. When meeting someone new at a party we would not cross-examine them with a series of closed questions such as 'Are you an estate agent?' 'Do you work in the city?' We would start with an open question such as 'What do you do?' or 'Tell me about yourself'. Some doctors seem to lose these skills when they enter the consulting room and feel the need to close their questions and limit the replies. Patients are also used to doctors working in this way and collude with this stilted mode of communication. When a doctor wishes to change styles, there is learning both for the doctor and for the patients.

Discovering the patient's agenda plays a fundamental part in producing an effective outcome for both doctor and patient. Virtually every patient in primary care will have had some thoughts about his condition and some ideas about what may need to be done about it, even though he might not be used to expressing his thoughts and opinions to his doctor. The doctor, often driven by the need to collect facts and meet the demands of protocols, is liable to concentrate on a limited, doctor-centred agenda. Yet, it is possible to gather the appropriate facts about the patient's symptoms and stick to a protocol using patient-centred skills. Asking open questions about clinical symptoms yields most of the answers required. After a patient has related his story, the doctor can easily check out facts that may have been missed and clarify the picture. This often takes less time than a barrage of closed questions. Beckman and Frankel (1984) in their study of consultations noted that the average time that a doctor waited before interrupting the patient was only 19 s. He went on to observe that if the doctor waited and encouraged the patient to speak, most patients could tell their story, their ideas, concerns and expectations, within 2 min.

Preparation: a supportive environment

The environment of a general practice consultation is often not conducive to facilitating change and development. Having too many patients and insufficient time to see them, puts most GPs under pressure. The consulting room is often too busy, and the session too frequently interrupted by colleagues and phone calls. In this case, the problems of practice management are disturbing the doctor, in addition to any personal issues that compete for concentration.

Problems of practice management that hinder the consultation need to be addressed. Booking times may need to be reviewed; it is possible that longer consultation times would make keeping to time easier. Staff may need clearer instructions as to when and when not to interrupt the consultation by phone or in person. If a doctor is to consult well, it will be helpful to know that everything possible has been done to aid concentration, particularly if he or she is wanting to try new approaches and have the time to reflect on them. This is a theme to which we will return later in the chapter.

Action: learning new skills

Skills development goes through predictable stages:

◆ setting clear objectives to be achieved
◆ setting explicit and realistic goals
◆ making opportunities to practise new skills
◆ getting feedback.

The tasks described in Chapter 6 could form the objectives to be achieved. Other objectives or schemes, such as those of Neighbour (1987), Stewart (1995), or Silverman *et al.* (1996) would function as well. The important factor here, is to be clear about what one is trying to do, and specific objectives are much more helpful than generalized objectives. For example, it is more effective

---

Box 8.2   **Learning new skills**

Action	Example
Divide the change planned into small manageable amounts, and make one change at a time	Start asking the patients their ideas and concerns about their symptoms and what they would like you to do for them
Be comfortable with one new skill before starting another	When that feels comfortable you can encourage joint decision making
Make a written plan for yourself at the beginning and the end of each surgery. Mentally review each consultation to see what was achieved	Plan: This surgery I will check each patient's understanding of the medicines I prescribe
Practice a new consultation skill at times when there are not so many pressures	It would be unwise to try out a new skill on a Friday night loaded with fit-in appointments. If it takes more time, book in longer time for a while
Continue to practise a skill until it no longer feels awkward. Change the words you use until they feel natural	If you do not like 'What do you think is wrong with you?' then try 'Have you any ideas what might be causing this?' or 'What might have started this off?'
Do not be put off by the patient's initial reaction. It is probably new for them too, and they might need some explanation	'I was asking because some people might be worried about symptoms like this and I wondered if you were'

---

to say 'I am going to discover exactly why each of my patients has come to see me today' than 'I am going to be more patient-centred'.

Establishing clear and specific objectives makes it easier to identify the skills that are needed. This may be accomplished either through reflection on everyday skills that are applicable to the consultation, or through reading the contributions of a number of authors on consultation skills cited in earlier chapters. Whatever the route to skills identification, experimentation and practice are required to incorporate those skills into the doctor's repertoire.

These stages can be incorporated into a plan such as the one set in Box 8.2.

Action: dealing with stress

Consulting with patients can be stressful. Changing the way one consults and doing something that is unfamiliar can add to that stress. It is important to consider how this stress can be managed. Roger Neighbour (1987) described the importance of recognizing and reducing stress in and around the consultation. He called this housekeeping, and described four approaches that can be considered:

1. *Reduce the cause*—identify and reduce the sources of the stress, for example, reduce waiting time for patients and stop unnecessary interruptions to the consultation.

2. *Improve coping skills*—Develop skills and resources to reduce the impact of stress e.g. improve consulting skills, make consulting easier and more satisfying for the doctor.

3. *Change attitude to stress*—Stress is not inevitably caused by stressors, it is a matter of perception. One way of alleviating stress is to change one's perception of the same events from negative to positive: from 'It's so awful that I have only 10 min with this patient' to 'I have 10 min with this patient and I'm going to make the best use of it I can.'

4. *Reduce the stress reaction*—When the stress arises in the consulting room the recognition of the signs of stress can in themselves reduce the tension. Muscle relaxation and controlled breathing can help to shed the worst sensations of tension. Taking a 'mini-break' or a walk, talking to someone, or taking a cup of coffee may all help.

In Chapter 5 we recognized that some patients produce emotional reactions in doctors. Some create positive feelings of satisfaction or pleasure, and others negative feelings of sadness or frustration. Naturally, there is a range of emotions in-between, and all patients will produce some kind of emotional response. The key is to use and benefit from the good responses, while diminishing and disregarding the bad. We have found it helpful to recognize and take ownership of the emotions. They are, after all, *our* emotions. This stops us blaming external factors for our feelings, either good or bad.

Taking ownership brings our emotions more under our control, encouraging us to reproduce the situations that we find positive. We might find that reflecting on achievements in the consultation makes us feel good. Patients might have stopped smoking or reduced alcohol consumption with our help; they might have been grateful for our input to a difficult relationship problem; we may have made an early diagnosis or a swift and timely referral. Individual doctors gain satisfaction from different factors. It is worth becoming aware of the factors that make us feel good so that we can reflect on them, and feel good, at will.

The doctor can work with this idea by keeping a very brief reflective diary of some of the positive emotions that have been experienced in the consulting room. It can help reproduce those situations at will. After the consultation, the doctor can check how effective he or she was by asking the ten questions in the Box 8.3. This feedback is often rewarding and the occasional bad experience is put into proportion.

Box 8.3 **How effective was I?**

1. Do I know significantly more about them than before the consultation?
2. Did I discover what mattered to them?
3. Did I listen?
4. Did I explore their agenda, beliefs and expectations?
5. Did I make an acceptable working diagnosis?
6. Did I use what they thought when I started explaining?
7. Did I share options for investigations or treatments?
8. Did I involve them in decision-making?
9. Did I make some attempt to check that they really understood?
10. Was I facilitative?

Doctors have bad days. They are as prone to illness or excesses as anyone else, and they can perform under par as a consequence. These human issues are common but they interfere with the effectiveness of the consultation and can jeopardize the relationship with the patient. So, what, if anything, can be done about it?

The first stage is awareness of the problem, and an admission that it is happening. This may not be easy when the issue is acute. A supportive working environment is an essential starting place. Later in this chapter we will be looking at the environment of the consultation and how it can become both patient-centred and supportive for the doctors and staff. Doctors can also develop the skills to monitor their feelings and may even conduct a brief 'mood check' at the start of each surgery so that remedial action can be taken when necessary.

Action: dealing with patients in new ways

One of the effects of a more open patient-centred consulting style is that patients reveal more of their problems and emotions. This can be a positive experience in which the doctor acquires new insights into his patient, and the patient feels better understood. On the other hand, it may cause the doctor's heart to sink, particularly if he or she does not have a sufficiently broad repertoire of psychological skills and resources to deal with the problem. In this case, the doctor may wish that the can of worms had never been opened.

It is extremely helpful to be able to discuss the patients that cause doctors difficulty. Constructive discussions produce improved outcomes for doctors and patients alike. This system dates back to the 1950s when Michael Balint set up the original discussion groups for doctors to discuss their patients. It continues today and may take the form of case discussion groups or critical incident analysis, both for principals and GP registrars. In some practices patients who are seen to cause all the doctors difficulty are shared out evenly and overtly among the doctors with help and support offered between colleagues. It can help to be able to discuss these difficult patients with even one sympathetic colleague: it can share the burden and create insight and new suggestions.

The doctors in a practice may have a view about a group of patients who are seen to be more difficult or demanding than others. We came across such an example during a practice visit. There was a feeling in the practice that a group of patients from a particular ethnic background were more demanding and difficult than others. The practice was encouraged to examine and measure the factors that were causing concern. They mapped the population; looked at consultation rates; looked at chronic disease incidence; measured missed appointment rates and compared them with another part of their population. None of the differences was significant except for the higher incidence of some diseases. This was an issue that they tackled by employing an interpreter, working with the leaders of that community and setting up a special chronic disease clinic. The practice felt proud of their achievement: they were recognized as a centre of excellence and the 'problem population' no longer produced the feelings that they had done previously.

Generally, doctors in practice need to match their skills with the dominant needs of the practice population. Those practitioners with many young families, whose surgeries are full of mothers and children presenting together, might gain new insights by learning about family therapy. The doctor who feels burdened by depressed or anxious patients might benefit from learning the strategies and skills of cognitive behavioural therapy or counselling. The doctor with a high workload of sexual problems might benefit from learning the techniques of brief sexual therapy.

Maintenance: outcomes for the doctor

If new behaviours are not rewarded they will not be maintained. How do we know how well we are doing in our consultations and reward ourselves for success? Feedback can be very haphazard for a doctor. Patients are often reluctant to be honest with their doctor for fear of upsetting them. Useful feedback needs to be elicited directly, and in a way that assists patients to be honest, producing information that can be used to increase the doctor's effectiveness.

Feedback in the consultation

The skills required to evaluate whether our tasks have been achieved are seldom seen in consultations but, if used, would enhance the consultation for the patient and the doctor. We first need to identify the patient's expectations and define clearly what the patient would like from the consultation. This includes the medical outcomes, the emotional outcomes and the process of the consultation. These are some of the patient-centred benchmarks of an effective consultation. The sort of questions that might be helpful are: 'You said when you came you were concerned that you might have caught something. How do you feel now?' 'You were feeling very low, how are you feeling now?' 'Have I helped with your wish to stop smoking?'. Different doctors will develop questions to suit their own style.

There are substantial advantages to seeking feedback in the consultation. First, if the doctor has missed something, it can be corrected. Second, it helps the doctor to identify in the consultation those things that work and produce a good reaction. With good record keeping, feedback may be obtained in a subsequent consultation, enhancing continuity of care, and collecting more thoughtful feedback in hindsight.

Feedback beyond the consultation

One of the easiest and most useful methods for obtaining feedback outside the consultation is to use a patient questionnaire. Many have been published and are readily available. 'Ask The Patient' is available from the College of Health. There is the General Practice Assessment Survey (Greco 1998) and the Patient Enablement Instrument (Howie *et al.* 1998), to name but three. These instruments have all been validated and contain published ranges of previous results for comparison. They are easily obtainable and most are easy to use. The alternative is to develop a tailored questionnaire in the practice, but these frequently lead to uninterpretable results and frustration after a great deal of work. For this reason, we recommend that a validated questionnaire is used, at least initially.

To obtain qualitative feedback from a more specific group, some doctors will convene a group of patients for a discussion about their care. Examples might be a group of patients who have had a recent heart attack, or patients with diabetes that is looked after in the practice's diabetic clinic. This is a focus group and can help in planning the service to particular care groups.

The environment

The environment in which a doctor works can make a great deal of difference to the effectiveness of the consultation. There are environments that can make the doctor's life easier and enable her to maximize her skills with patients or hinder effectiveness by disruptions, by unconducive surroundings or unhelpful systems. Mrs Hall's consultation is a case in point:

> The waiting room is full because the doctor is running 40 min late. The receptionist is frazzled because there are no more available appointments and yet the phone is constantly ringing. Mrs. Hall hears the buzzer and the light flashes next to Dr Warden's name but she is unsure if she is next. 'Of course you are' the receptionist exclaims 'the doctor is waiting for you now.'
>
> On entering the consulting room the doctor looks up and says 'Good morning Mrs. Jones'. After explaining who she is, Dr Warden calls for Mrs. Hall's records and spends a moment updating himself about her case. This is a little

difficult because the letters are jumbled and the record cards are not in date order. The doctor looks up and says, 'How can I help you?' Mrs. Hall starts describing the abdominal pains that she has had for the last two months but her story is interrupted by the phone ringing. It is the receptionist who says, 'Dr. Warden, you asked Mr Evans to phone back to discuss his blood test result and he is on the phone now' 'Excuse me' the Doctor says to Mrs. Hall, and leaves her waiting while he explained the results of a raised PSA to Mr Evans. 'Sorry about that, you were telling me about your bowels' 'No doctor, I was describing my periods relating to this pain in my tummy'.

Many of the systems in doctors' practices are run with the doctors and staff in mind and not the patients. Doctors are frequently busy so the booking system is designed to plug any gaps in the doctor's time: it does not matter if patients are kept waiting. On their part, patients are so grateful to see a doctor that they do not mind waiting for a long time to see one. Some doctors try to do two jobs at a time, consulting with one patient in the room and another on the phone. This perception by some in the health service, that doctors' time is in some way more valuable than any one else's can lead to systems that are profession-centred and not patient-centred.

Patient-centred culture

For a practice to maintain systems that produce high patient satisfaction, the culture of the practice needs to be patient focused. In such a practice, the members will enjoy contact with patients; they will try to please the patients at each opportunity; they will speak well of patients when they talk amongst them-selves; they will seek patients' views of the practice, constantly trying to improve the service. This state is difficult both to achieve and to sustain; most fall short, but seeking it raises staff and doctor morale.

The partners and practice manager need to agree that they are going to create a patient-centred culture, and they need to ascertain their current state. A patient survey as described above may be a very good starting point. Front line staff often have good ideas about what the patients appreciate and where there are problems. The culture of putting the patient first, listening to patients and staff, and continuously trying to improve the service requires leadership to become firmly established.

The culture of the practice stems primarily from how the doctors treat the patients and how they talk about their patients to other members of the primary health care team. This 'internal talk' from the doctors governs how the other members of the practice think about the patients and that, in turn, influences their behaviour with the patients. If the doctors explain to their staff the reasons behind their patients' behaviour, encouraging them to understand the patient's journey through the health care system, the staff will be more understanding of the difficulties the patients encounter. This can be instigated in a staff education

session or as a series of one-to-one meetings with staff members. The importance of 'internal talk' cannot be overemphasized. The complaints procedure can
be used as a method to review change, even though complaints usually cause a lot
of upset. Similarly, letters of thanks and congratulations can be circulated through
the practice to celebrate successes and to foster a climate of appreciation.

Sometimes one doctor in a practice wishes to change but others are reluctant
to do so. It is possible to instigate changes in one doctor's personal approach to
practice but very difficult to maintain the enthusiasm required. It is easy to
revert to previous habits. Often with genuine involvement and discussion, it is
possible to gain allies within the practice. Fellow professionals who see patient
care in the same way will join in, trying to bring about similar changes. The
more the number of team members who wish to practise in a patient-centred
way, the easier it is to change the culture of the practice for all.

There are many opportunities in the practice for developing a patient-centred
culture. It is possible to include *consulting* in the clinical governance plan for
the practice. As part of the continuing professional development in the practice,
some are reviewing their consultations with each other. With established criteria, some groups of doctors share a videotape of their consultations and get
feedback from their colleagues. This is part of the doctors' personal learning
and tends to be included in their personal development plans.

Many practices have practice meetings and these can be developed to include
training sessions on phone answering, problem solving, greeting etc. Some
practices have away-days together to plan new systems and develop the care in
the practice. Practices also benefit from the opportunity to learn from others
whether it be on courses or in meetings, or by participating in reciprocal visits.

Appointments and time/work pressure

One of the most inhibiting factors on an effective consultation is time. The time
that the patient has to wait to get an appointment; the time waiting in the queue
to see the doctor; and time pressures on the doctor to complete the consultation,
all put pressure on both the doctor and the patient and can reduce their ability to
get the best out of each other. Many booking systems, both in hospital and in
general practice, are not designed to bring together the doctor and patient at the
same time, in the same place, feeling relaxed and ready to work together. They
tend to be set up to maximize throughput and efficiency, with little regard for
effectiveness or for the doctor's preferred working pace.

Booked appointments may be seven and a half minutes long but the doctor
may need 10 min for each patient to consult, make notes and take phone calls.
Day after day, week after week, the doctor sees the last patient in the surgery
about 50 min late. The patients become irritated, feeling slighted by the assumed
lack of respect for them and their time. The doctor increasingly feels harassed.
This is no way for any consultation to start. The problem would be solved if the

receptionist were to increase the booking time to 10 min. The doctor would finish at the *same* time as he always has, and the patients would not build up tension in the waiting room. Consultations would begin with both parties feeling more relaxed.

Some practices have matched capacity with demand, and made their appointment systems patient-centred. In this way, they have also been able to reduce the delay in getting an appointment to see a doctor. The practices have counted the total number of patients seen in a typical day or week, and also the number of appointments provided in the same period. Appointments have then been provided to meet the assessed need with the aim of ensuring that most patients are seen by a doctor within 24 h. In this way, they have improved the working lives of their doctors and the satisfaction of their patients. Further information on this theme can be found in the United Kingdom from the National Primary Care Collaborative (www.npdt.org) and in the United States, from the Institute for Health Improvement (www.ihi.org).

Even when the appointment system is running well, a few delays inevitably occur. Some of these are common but unpredictable, such as discovering an urgent medical condition or a patient who needs more time. Most patients understand and tolerate these unavoidable delays, provided they are exceptional. The frustration comes when the patient does not know the cause or the probable length of the delay. An empathic receptionist can keep the patients informed and reduce these tensions in the practice, provided he or she remains within the bounds of patient confidentiality.

Call systems

Many doctors' practices have grown over the years. If a person does not understand the call system, or gets lost within the building, they will finally arrive at the consulting room irritated and anxious. Care needs to be taken to design these systems with patients in mind.

Record systems and computers

Record systems are becoming more complicated and sophisticated. They require to be computerized, and yet it is difficult to maintain these records on the computer and to consult in a patient-centred way. Inevitably, the need to enter and retrieve information on the computer disrupts the consultation. There are helpful steps that can be taken to minimize this disruption, however.

Before the consultation, it is useful to look at the computer and/or the notes gathering the relevant information to minimize the use of the records during the consultation. This task is made much easier if the information is easily retrievable. Paper records in order, an accurate summary sheet of important clinical details, an accurate prescription list and the use of flow charts in the notes, can make this task quick and straightforward. Most good computer systems now make the process of finding data from records much easier.

It does require a certain amount of discipline to enter accurate data at each consultation, and from hospital letters received, in order to maintain the quality and usefulness of the records. In order to prevent data entry disrupting the consultation, it is important to distinguish between the information that needs to go on the computer during the consultation, and that which can be entered when the patient has left.

Summary

1. Arguably, the most important determinant of doctors' health and job satisfaction is the extent to which he or she is in control of his or her own life and work.

2. Enabling patients to increase that sense of control, and to acquire the ability to make changes in their lives, is one of our core aims for our consultations.

3. This chapter has aimed to help doctors take control and make changes in their work, with the hope and expectation that it will improve their health and job satisfaction as well.

9 Teaching in educational settings

The ability of doctors to communicate with their patients has long been recognized as essential for the practice of medicine. More recently, however, there has been a growing recognition that some styles of communication are more effective than others. That effective communication can be taught and learned, and that the ability to communicate should be assessed as part of the assessment of clinical competence for medical students and doctors.

Undergraduate teaching

The consensus statement issued after the International Conference on Communication in Toronto in 1991 (Simpson *et al.* 1991) summarized the evidence about effective information, current deficiencies in practice and proven methods of teaching. In 1993, the General Medical Council (1993) recommended that communication skills should be taught throughout the education of medical students in the United Kingdom, and similar statements have been made by the Association of American Medical Colleges (1998) regarding medical education in the United States and Canada.

The last published survey in 1998 of communication skills teaching reported considerable progress, but also great variability, in UK medical schools (Hargie *et al.* 1998). The ways in which this has been implemented varies greatly, with some medical schools providing skills teaching away from clinical settings, often by general practitioners, psychiatrists, or behavioural scientists. Others have been able to integrate communication skills within their clinical teaching, and to include it in the assessment of their students. Most medical schools use a combination of small group teaching, role-play with simulated patients, and video-feedback.

There is also a growing consensus amongst teachers of communication skills about the requirements for the development and implementation of communication skills teaching, and a statement of these was published in 1999 (Makoul and Schofield 1999). The most important of these is the need to integrate communication skills teaching with other clinical teaching, particularly history taking, and to involve clinical teachers both as role models and advocates for patient-centred consulting.

Communication teachers in medical schools in the United Kingdom have also developed a core curriculum which is derived from the needs of junior hospital doctors (Schofield T, personal communication). It includes not only patient-centred interviewing, but also communication in special situations such as breaking bad news and communication with people of different backgrounds and cultures. It takes a broad view of communication to embrace team-working skills, communication with colleagues and assertiveness. It also considers the attitudes and values that are required, and need to be fostered in medical students to enable them to be patient-centred whilst surviving the pressures of working as a doctor. However, there remains great variation in the extent to which this curriculum has been implemented in different medical schools.

The challenge for postgraduate education, including training for general practice, is that these differences between medical schools produces great variations in experience and ability of their graduates. The consequence is that any programme of further communication skills teaching must be able to respond very flexibly to the needs of individuals.

Vocational training for general practice

Over the last 20 years in the United Kingdom, there has been a great deal of progress in all the Deaneries regarding the development of learning and teaching on the consultation. This activity in most cases pre-dated the inclusion of the consultation in the Membership of the Royal College of General Practitioners (MRCGP) and summative assessment but this change has concentrated many minds. Some Directors of General Practice and their adviser teams have developed a Deanery strategy and the supporting structures and processes to implement it. The example of this in the Oxford Deanery is a strategy produced in 1993 stating:

1. Each trainee should have regular, systematic training, and feedback on their own consultations in their practice.

2. Innovations in this field should be considered.

3. The programme should be evaluated.

This meant there were implications for various groups in the Deanery:

1. The Trainers and Training Practices needed equipment, skills, knowledge of the literature, and practice management procedures to cope with videoing consultations.

2. The Course Organizers needed to gain the knowledge and skills to teach on the theoretical background of effective consulting.

3. The Trainers Groups needed to develop trainers' consulting and teaching skills using their own videos and pre-recorded tutorial videos as part of their regular group programme.

4. The Advisers team needed to encourage a consistent message and practice in the Registrar Introductory Course, the Trainers' Course, in the selection and re-selection of trainers, and in the Registrars' assessment of the practice.

They also needed to ensure that suitable training was available for all, and that there was a uniform approach to the issue of informed consent to video recording in the practices, and to handling matters of confidentiality.

Initially the Deanery provided suitable video equipment that circulated around the schemes within the region but, once the value of the technique was seen, most of the training practices bought their own machines. A survey of the training practices of the Oxford Deanery in 1994 showed that 97 per cent of training practices had easy access to video recording equipment and 61 per cent of trainees observed and were taught on their consultations more than four times in their trainee year (Havelock, personal communication).

Training the trainers

The Deanery supports the strategy that the training practice is the important place for the Registrar to obtain most of their teaching on the consultation. To support the trainers in those skills, we run the Trainers Consultation Workshop 'Consulting with Challenging Patients: Learning and Teaching'.

The course is based on the theoretical basis discussed in Chapter 7 and works on three main principles about doctors:

1. Doctors have a wider role in the consultation than just the diagnosis and management of disease, such as health promotion, modifying health seeking behaviour and encouraging patient autonomy.
2. Nearly all doctors have a range of sophisticated communication skills: though these are sometimes not used in the consultation.
3. Everyone can improve his or her communication skills.

The consultation skills workshop

*   Day One
    (a) theoretical input and skills demonstration;
    (b) discussion and definition of challenging patients;
    (c) using tutors' consultations.
*   Day Two
    (a) consultation feedback and teaching demonstration;
    (b) using simulated patients.
*   Day Three
    (a) teaching practice and feedback;
    (b) Using videotaped consultations with real patients.

Day 1

We begin by establishing the participants' previous experience of communication skills teaching, their own expectations of the course and what they wish to achieve. We also ask about those patients the learners find challenging to deal with as doctors. The issues around those challenging patients are then discussed and collated for discussion in the large group. These discussions take place in small groups of up to six doctors and the groups aim to meet these individual needs through the course. This deliberately parallels the process of patient-centred consulting and learner-centred teaching that the workshop aims to promote.

We then present the evidence and rationale that underpins our approach to the consultation and also describe other approaches to analysing and teaching the consultation that the trainers may wish to explore and use. We give specific evidence and help for the issues that have come out of the participants' own difficulties with patients. Subsequently we describe and rehearse the process of observing, describing and giving feedback on consultations using the tutors' tapes as examples. Thus, by the end of the first day, the participants have experienced a model of what we are trying to teach both for the consultation and for consultation teaching.

Day 2

The second day is spent in small groups with each member of the group in turn conducting a consultation with a simulated patient in front of the group and then receiving feedback from them. This has a number of functions:

1. The group has the opportunity to rehearse the process of observing and giving feedback on consultations and the group leader can participate in the process, helping group members develop their skills during the day.
2. Individual doctors have the opportunity to experience what it is like to receive feedback from colleagues and to learn from it.
3. By explicitly identifying effective skills and strategies in each consultation, the group members have the opportunity to learn a wider repertoire of effective consultation behaviours so that, in their subsequent teaching, they are able to offer their learners alternative approaches rather than just their own.

The simulated patients play a very important part in the day and have been trained in the teaching technique they use. First, they act patient roles that can be chosen to provide a variety of teaching points. We ask them, where appropriate, to role-play some of the patients the learners described as challenging on day one. Second, they give feedback in the group *in role* thus providing feedback from the 'patient' in the role-play. Third, they come out of role and provide feedback as co-teachers drawing on their previous experience of consulting with hundreds of doctors.

Day 3

On the third day each member of the group is invited to watch a pre-recorded consultation by another member of the group and then to give feedback to that doctor. The rest of the group do not participate in feedback to the doctor but instead observe the teaching and give feedback to the teacher on its effectiveness. This means that each member of the group has the opportunity to rehearse as an individual what they learned in the group on the previous day. The workshop thus demonstrates the three features of effective skills teaching by providing:

◆ an explicit model of what is to be learned
◆ opportunities for practice
◆ observation and feedback.

Finally the members of the course are invited to write a personal action plan of how they intend to use and develop what they have learned during the course, before they evaluate the programme.

This workshop is supported by work carried out in the monthly trainers' group in each of the nine Vocational Training (VT) Schemes. The groups:

◆ look at video tapes of the trainers and teach on them
◆ describe and use different teaching methods on the consultation, for example, Roger Neighbour's approach, Interpersonal Process Recall (IPR), The Cambridge-Calgary method
◆ discuss videotaped tutorials
◆ discuss cases that have implications for teaching
◆ discuss Registrar teaching and the use of the video.

The trainer's skills of teaching on a consultation are assessed on three-yearly training practice assessments by looking at real videotapes of both consulting with patients and teaching the Registrar.

Courses for registrars

Each of the Registrars within the Deanery are invited to attend a two day residential course 'The Registrar Introductory Course' and here they are introduced to the concepts of effective consulting, methods of teaching, and planning their education throughout the year. The session uses their experiences of being patients or those experiences of a close relative, this highlights the need for patient-centred consulting. Although the main emphasis of learning the consultation is in the practice, many of the VT schemes will include group sessions on the day release course that approach the issue from different perspectives, such as:

◆ peer discussion of videotapes of their consultations
◆ journal review of the evidence for effective consulting

- discussion with patient groups about consulting
- audits of patient satisfaction questionnaires
- case discussion of 'difficult patients' (Balint Group)
- discussions about ethical issues that affect consultations
- discussion of patient narratives
- introduction of new strategies and skills, for example Cognitive Behavioural Therapy, Family Therapy, Psychosexual Counselling.

Unsurprisingly, we have found that Registrars get a more coherent view of effective consulting when there is greater co-ordination between the teaching on the day-release course and the teaching in the practice.

Teaching in practice

The trainer needs to change and develop their teaching on the consultation to meet the developing need of the Registrar. We have developed guidance for a stepwise and developmental approach.

Week 1

When the Registrar comes to the practice they are often straight out of an SHO post where the concentration was on gathering as much evidence from a patient as possible as quickly as possible—and surviving! Patient-centred consulting is rarely encouraged within a busy hospital job, so we first have to take the learner through the theory behind effective consulting, its evidence base, and the values that underpin a patient-centred approach.

Because it is difficult to change many behaviours at once it is better to concentrate on one aspect at a time. We start with the role of patients' ideas in an effective consultation.

As we mentioned above, the process needs:

- an understanding of what is to be achieved
- how it is to be achieved
- practice and feedback.

When this has been achieved then the Registrar can concentrate on, for example, 'sharing understanding',—the evidence for it, the skills needed, practice and feedback, until it is established in the doctor's consulting repertoire. The subsequent stages of shared decision-making, involving the patient in decision making and managing risk factors all follow when earlier skills have been learned and are regularly used. The regular use of the video camera and the analysis of consultations is essential for the registrar to gain these skills and get feedback on his/her progress.

This stepwise process can start very early in a Registrar year so that these skills develop in parallel with new clinical skills. To aid the learning other approaches to the consultation can be used and developed, such as Roger Neighbour's 'connecting' and the importance of the patient's opening gambit.

Learning effective consulting takes time: time for teaching and looking at videos and time within the Registrar's consultations to practise these new techniques. It is therefore important that the Registrar maintains a long consultation time for much of the year because it is much more difficult to learn new skills while under time pressure. The initial priority is to learn to consult effectively and only then to learn to consult at the required consulting speed. Once the consultations are effective and mostly contain the elements of patient-centred consulting, then the same teaching techniques can be used to help the registrar get up to speed. The skills of efficient use of time can be discussed and practiced: early identification of cues; active listening without interruption; guiding discussion; not repeating information without meaning to; checking understanding throughout the consultation; being prepared before a consultation and many others. The review of the videotapes can look at these skills while maintaining the effectiveness and new skills can be offered.

When the Registrar can consult effectively and is up to speed, they are ready to submit a videotape for MRCGP or Summative Assessment. Consultations for these assessments can be collected as the training develops and need be neither a major hurdle nor particularly time-consuming. This might happen, with the right approach to teaching, as early as four months through the Registrar year.

Learning on the consultation continues after the external tests of competency have been taken and passed. The summative assessment and MRCGP pass are minimum standards. We advocate career-long learning in effective consulting to enhance the patient's experience in the consulting room. The doctor can pass the MRCGP, for example, without mastering such patient-centred behaviours as seeking patients' ideas and concerns, checking patients' understanding, involving patients in management decisions, or explaining in the patient's own terms. These are doctor behaviours that have been shown to produce better outcomes for the patient so further development of these is essential.

In addition to the basic skills, the Registrar learns skills from other professionals such as counselling, family therapy, sexual therapy, and the like. This would involve further reading, sitting in with the appropriate professional, practising the skills, and getting feedback, maybe the registrar might wish to gain skills in cognitive behavioural therapy and seek a course or find further reading. The Registrar could also carry out an audit on patient satisfaction or patient feedback on consultations. The consultation and clinical communication might be an area that a highflying Registrar might also wish to research further.

Junior/senior hospital settings

This is a developing area and an area that is ripe for development. In the United Kingdom, most of the work on consultation development has been in primary care though there are several notable exceptions. Hospital doctors often need a different approach to learning consultation skills than do general practitioners and GP Registrars. There are obvious differences of context, for example, the clinic or ward setting. Other subtler differences such as the feeling of time pressure, and the culture of education that is not, in many places, as highly developed as in primary care. The education techniques therefore need to reflect those differences:

1. The timing and duration of the workshop need to reflect the work patterns of the participants. For example, Consultants seem to have difficulty devoting whole days to education.

2. The setting of the workshop needs to remove junior staff from the tyranny of their pagers. Usually this means that they have to be trained away from their hospital.

3. Examples of patients used in the role-play need to be tailored and totally credible to the doctor or the exercise is rejected.

4. Feedback has to be handled particularly sensitively and skilfully to counter the 'blame culture' often found within hospitals.

These are, of course, features that need considering for any educational event for any group of people but they have particular salience for hospital doctors. Similarly, there are other elements of the teaching that are always relevant to all doctors in training, such as presentation of the evidence base for effective consulting.

Workshops and courses for CME

Doctors frequently cite 'difficult consultations' as a primary cause of stress, though they tend to be reluctant to attend workshops that address those issues. They will attend lectures and ask questions but this form of education is unlikely to produce changes within the consultations and relieve those stresses.

We found it was possible to overcome many of these problems by providing a facilitator to work in the practices. The Wycombe Primary Care Prevention Project was set up in 1992 to help practices and practitioners develop their prevention and health promotion role. Part of this role, of course, is effective communication about health issues. To develop these skills we set up workshops that moved the participants through progressive learning on a subject, to the practical application of that subject within their practice and their consultations. This involved role-play and feedback of the consultation, with clear criteria and using structured feedback. Uptake rates among the general practitioners in the area were high and sustained.

Methods for learning skills

It can be very beneficial to develop consultation skills in a small group of trusted colleagues. This could be a young practitioners group, a CME group, or a partnership. The importance is to be clear about the purpose of the group, rules within which they will work, and sensitive, clear leadership. Often the local CME GP tutor can offer guidance and support.

We have found that a stepwise approach can be really helpful:

Step 1. Reduce working isolation
Consulting is an individual and personal activity. Few doctors share what goes on in the consulting room with anyone except the patient yet it is very much easier to learn more effective consulting with others of like mind. The other learners could be partners, peers, or other people in the Primary Health Care Team, who consult with patients. A great deal of successful learning can be multi disciplinary with health visitors, practice nurses, community psychiatric nurses, or any other professionals. Learning with even one other person can make a real difference.

Step 2. Decide what is needed in a consultation
This is the starting point of any development process: to define what is effective. For us, our task list serves this purpose, but there are alternatives to which we have often referred. The criteria need to be agreed, and the values implicit in them discussed until the group is sufficiently comfortable with them to proceed further. It can help encourage the group to think of the criteria from their perspective as patients or users of the health service, it encourages a more patient-centred frame of mind.

Step 3. Observe the consultation
When trying to improve consultations, it is important to be as specific as possible, and to think in terms of *each* consultation rather than consultations in general. To share consultations with others, the learner will either have to record it on video or audiotape, or invite direct observation by sitting in. Making a recording of the consultation is easier, more effective, and less disruptive for both doctor and patient, with the added advantage that the consulting doctor can also directly observe the process.

Step 4. Compare performances with set objectives

Step 5. Improving the less effective parts of the consultation

Step 6. Incorporate the changes into everyday practice
These steps are described above in the feedback section. The issues are the same for practising health professionals as they are for GP Registrars, but as

with hospital doctors (also described above) the hazards and difficulties need to be avoided by skilful and well considered teaching.

Clinical governance and the consultation

In the United Kingdom, the rapid pace of developments of such issues as clinical governance and revalidation make writing about them in 2002 difficult. Yet there is increasing recognition that effective consulting is an important quality issue for all doctors. Good Medical Practice (GMC 1999) contains many references to communication with patients. This has been taken up by the Royal College of General Practitioners document 'Good Medical Practice for General Medical Practitioners' and specific criteria have been laid down for excellent and unacceptable behaviour in the communication between doctor and patient. These criteria and standards, under the heading 'Professional Relationship with Patients: maintaining the trust', are likely to be used in the revalidation of doctors.

Summary

Every medical practitioner can improve their consulting skills with patients. In order to do so, they need:

- an explicit model of what is to be learned
- opportunities for practice
- observation and feedback.

10 Describing and assessing consultations

Introduction

This chapter will consider the large variety of ways in which a consultation can be described or assessed, and the basis on which to choose between them. Some approaches are entirely descriptive, while others include assessment against agreed criteria; some methods are comprehensive and include the whole consultation, others select particular aspects of interest; some are based on external observation, some on the views of the patient, and some are self-assessments by the doctor. The choice depends on one's purpose, which can be broadly divided into teaching, quality improvement, regulatory assessment, or research.

Teaching

In earlier chapters, a number of principles of effective teaching and learning were described. One is that skills can be acquired best from an explicit model of what is to be learned, opportunities to practice new skills, and from feedback. In this approach there is a clear link between what is to be learned and what is to be observed and assessed, and this is often expressed as some form of rating scale. The content should be appropriate to the stage of development of the learner. First year medical students, without a knowledge base, are unlikely to benefit from tools helpful to fourth and fifth year students. Doctors in vocational training (VT) will require more sophisticated assessments. Rating scales for students may include specific skills, while our approach to teaching practising doctors is to define tasks to be achieved, and to assess the individual's effectiveness at achieving them. For teaching it is much more appropriate that the content of the assessment is appropriate or valid, than whether or not it can be assessed reliably. Differences of opinion can be the starting point for valuable discussion, rather than a weakness of the assessment.

Another educational principle described earlier was the importance of developing self-awareness and reflective practice. It is therefore important to encourage learners to assess themselves, and to compare these assessments with the views of an external observer and with their patients. These assessments can include a discussion of thoughts and feelings at the time as well as the values that underpin the practice. The doctor's cycle, described in Chapter 2 is a framework for this type of assessment. The type of assessment used in learning and teaching is usually described as formative. This implies that the methodology will help in the development of improved consulting behaviour.

Quality improvement

There is a growing recognition of the need for doctors to continue to review their work, maintain and improve their standards and submit themselves to external scrutiny throughout their professional lifetime. The consultation is at the heart of medical practice and performance in the consultation must therefore be included in this process. Assessment methods may include self-assessment, peer review, and feedback from patients. Not only will doctors need to keep up with new medical knowledge, but to survive will need to develop new skills and attitudes to cope with changes in the doctor-patient relationship. The underlying purpose of consultation assessment at any stage of a doctor's career is to help increase understanding of the interpersonal processes that improve outcomes for patients and their doctors.

Regulatory assessment

Assessment drives learning. This is the best reason for end point assessment of consulting ability. There are other reasons, less developmental but important, such as protecting the public from poor communicators, maintaining professional standards and creating clear career hurdles allowing externally regulated professional progression, such as medical school finals to Membership of the Royal College of General Practitioners (MRCGP) or MRCP to FRCGP by assessment. Regulatory has often been referred to as summative assessment but in the United Kingdom this term (Summative Assessment) has been applied to a specific measurement of minimal clinical and consulting competence at the end of GP VT and is no longer useful as a generic term for that reason.

Regulatory assessments need to be appropriate to the stage of professional development at which they are administered, and to have a content that is related to the teaching that has been received. They also have to be able to discriminate between good and poor performance, and do this in a way that is fair and reliable.

Regulatory assessments are designed to *discriminate* between candidates, and this is related to the purpose of the assessment. A measure designed to assess minimal competence, at which 95 per cent will be expected to pass, is going to be a different tool from that which seeks to measure optimal competence at a particular stage of apprenticeship, say allowing 70 per cent to progress through. A later career measure such as Fellowship might reasonably anticipate a 50 per cent pass rate.

Research

Research into the consultation has been both qualitative and quantitative. A review of these approaches is beyond the scope of this book. Suffice to say that qualitative approaches seek to understand what is going on in the consultation usually with few pre-conceptions, while quantitative research may also be descriptive, but may also seek to test specific hypotheses. Many research instruments therefore assess selective aspects of the consultation relevant to the hypothesis under study. They are also required to do this reliably.

Factors in the choice of an assessment instrument

The words validity and reliability have already entered into this discussion. As well as these, the issues of feasibility and acceptability will also enter into the choice of an approach to assessment, and in teaching and regulation one can also be concerned about the educational impact of the method. These issues will now be considered in more detail.

Validity

Validity is a complex issue and the arguments about it can get very academic. We will try to highlight the important concepts as they relate to the different reasons for assessment. Validity is concerned with two fundamental questions: the extent to which an assessment instrument or method actually measures what it is designed to measure; and how well does it correlate with other measures of the same thing. We offer three main areas of validity with important subdivisions.

Evidence for validity can come from a number of sources. Some involve the opinion of experts in the field; others require the collection of further data, to be used in an empirical validation; yet others involve the investigation of patterns of performance within a controlled setting or an examination. The notion of *'face' validity*, meaning 'this looks sensible and relates to real issues' is widely used, but is often little more than a question of 'does this look OK?'

Content validity is the extent to which the content of the instrument or assessment reflects the range of knowledge, skills, or behaviours that are to be assessed, in the situations in which these are required. For example, a first year medical student could be assessed on their questioning and listening skills when interviewing a "normal" patient, while a final year student could be assessed breaking bad news or explaining treatment to patients and obtaining informed consent. The performance on a small number of similar items will be better correlated than performance on a larger number of different attributes. For example, a doctor may be very good at explaining, but less effective dealing with emotions and displaying empathy. There may therefore be a trade off between the content validity of a measure and its internal consistency.

Another aspect of content validity might be the extent to which the evidence of competence which the assessor collects is representative of the generality of performance. This is a question both of sampling and of fidelity. We will return to this debate later in the chapter but the assessment of a doctor's consulting abilities using indirect methodologies such as role play and simulation can be seen to have a different type of content validity from assessment of directly observed 'real' behaviour using video. The simulation may be a valid test of competence but an inference of subsequent performance may be questionable, similarly a valid direct assessment of performance cannot be used to generalize about competence.

Criterion validity is the correlation between the item assessed and other measures of the same attribute. Criterion validity is usually divided into two constructs: *concurrent validity*, comparing different methodologies measuring the same criterion, and *predictive validity*, determining whether the assessment of the consulting criteria will predict subsequent outcomes? Concurrent validity is used to compare new assessments with established assessments, or with some gold standard. For example, Howie *et al.* (1998) compared their new enablement measure with other established measures of patient satisfaction to establish its concurrent validity. The next stage to measure predictive validity would be to establish that patients who feel more enabled have improved health outcomes.

Construct validity is one of the most difficult to establish. The question is how does the assessment relate to our hypotheses or constructs about what we are assessing? For example, if we are setting out to assess competent consulting, our assessment should be able to distinguish apprentices from masters. To a large extent, competence in consulting is acquired over time and is expected to bear a close relationship to experience for the majority of doctors. This is probably not a linear relationship, for there may come a point at which increasing experience implies declining competence. If we are assessing the patient centredness of a consultation, does our assessment correlate with measures of outcomes for patients? (Stewart 1995). Construct validity is established by a series of studies which can confirm the hypotheses, but can be brought into question by a single study that refutes it.

Where it has been possible to gather evidence for the validity for our approach, the evidence has been positive. Validity is a demanding concept that goes beyond asking a lot of people if they think you are doing the right thing.

Reliability

Reliability appears to be a simple concept: the extent to which one can rely on the result of an assessment to measure accurately the item to be assessed. For example, a single measurement of blood pressure may vary for many reasons including fluctuations in the blood pressure itself (subject variation), measurement errors in the machine used to take the pressure, differences between the same observer at different times (intra-observer variation), or between different observers (inter-observer variation). Reliability can be increased by such steps as repeated measures, increasing the precision of the criteria for the assessment, multiple observers, and assessor training.

If a rating scale has multiple items, it is possible to establish the correlation between the scores for each item, and a number of methods for this have been developed (Streiner and Norman 1995). Low levels of correlation would suggest that the scores vary randomly and have little to do with each other; high levels of correlation mean that some of the items may be redundant.

Human communication is complex and it is often the subtleties that make the difference. Achieving good reliability while measuring what really matters is not an easy task, many assessments fall at this hurdle. Reliability is most important for regulatory assessment. Careers are on the line. In this case an important element of reliability is the repeatability of the instrument, so that it generates similar results from cohort to cohort.

Generalizability is a related concept, affecting such decisions as how many consultations need to be watched to form a reliable judgement. There are two issues here. The first is whether the performance observed on a single occasion is representative of usual performance: the good or bad day phenomenon. The second is the extent that one can safely generalize from performance in one area to other areas. The evidence is that doctors may have some skills but not others, and can handle some situations better than others. A reliable assessment depends on an adequate sample covering a range of skills and situations.

Feasibility

Regulatory and research assessments are most affected by this consideration. For example, a 20 station simulated surgery may have high reliability but the logistics of running such an examination for say 1500 candidates a year are massively complex without an efficient and large organization behind it. A similar project on a local basis for much smaller numbers may be possible. Research is frequently bedevilled by considerations of sample size, grants, time available, and so on, and most research is a compromise between aspirations and reality.

Acceptability

Assessments, to be effective, must be acceptable to all involved: the assessed, the assessors, and the patients. This is not easy to achieve. Assessing consulting performance, and so inferring the degree of competence displayed, is an emotive issue. No doctor wishes to be found wanting is this central area of his or her practice. This perceived threat is one reason for the oft-stated dislike of both formative and regulatory assessments. Those being assessed have to be convinced of the merits of the method before they will be prepared to subject themselves to it. Of course, if the assessment is imposed but seen to be flawed, this will generate considerable resentment, and a climate unconducive to improving consulting. In many regulatory consulting assessments, the assessors are doctors, performing this task on a voluntary basis. This means they have to be involved, feel committed to the process, and derive educational benefits from it, or else why would they do it?

In this new century, patients are rightly demanding a greater say in the regulation of doctors. Public opinion and the influence of pressure groups are driving the assessment processes. Consulting assessment methods that do not reflect the *mores* of our society will be seen as unacceptable. The inference is inescapable: patients must be involved in the derivation of consulting assessments.

Educational impact

For many reading this book, educational impact will be the most important consideration for a consulting assessment methodology. A good quality regulatory assessment will influence the learners and teachers agendas for the better at any stage in the medical voyage. The corollary is regrettably also true; a poor assessment will set back consulting development. It remains a challenge for all who care about the importance of good communication between doctor and patient that the educational impact of any assessment methodology should be positive. If the influence is deleterious in any way, if it is de-motivating, de-skilling, or perhaps too divisive, then the assessment must be modified or rejected.

We have argued throughout this book that doctors should deliberately seek their patients' perspectives and consult in a non-patronizing way that values involvement, and sharing. We have cited evidence that these behaviours are still unusual for most doctors and, in order to improve this situation for our patients, we would argue that all regulatory methods must contain assessment of such behaviours in order to drive the learning curriculum. This book is most concerned with teaching and learning, but the teaching and learning need to be assessed. Passing or failing exams that fulfil the above criteria must become an accepted part of the learning cycle.

Competence or performance: can or does?

There is a difference between that which the doctor knows how to do (can do), and that which the doctor actually puts into practice (does). This is the difference between competence and performance.

Does
Shows how
Knows how
Knows

Miller's pyramid of clinical competence (Miller 1990) can be used to illustrate this debate. In the model, the highest level is 'does'. This is how the doctor actually performs in the consulting room. To assess at this level requires some form of direct observation such as sitting in to observe, or a video recording of the doctor–patient encounter. This level is however often assessed by role-play or consulting simulations. These methodologies are inherently less authentic because they involve artificial and arranged clinical scenarios, but are very powerful formative tools. There is a difficulty with such methods when used for regulatory purposes, because of the leap of faith required to be convinced that competence demonstrated by such assessments actually translates into real performance.

Further down the pyramid the 'knows how' level is often assessed by face-to-face tutorials in formative assessments and by oral examinations in regulative assessments. Results from the MRCGP examination have clearly demonstrated that candidates 'know how' and espouse patient-centred consulting. But, whereas around 85 per cent espouse the idea, only around 10 per cent demonstrate it in their videotaped consultations.

The 'knows' level is usually assessed for formative and research purposes by questionnaires and rating scales. For regulatory purposes, it tends to be assessed by written examinations. A brief glance at the pyramid makes it unsurprising that results from written examinations correlate poorly with actual performance.

The simple rule is that, the greater the veracity required of the assessment instrument, the higher up the pyramid you have to go. Some would argue that the word veracity could be substituted with validity.

Examples in practice

Teaching

Many of the frameworks used for formative assessment in teaching are comprehensive models based on a coherent and explicit view of the content and purpose of the consultation. Their content varies more with the stage of professional development for which the framework was developed than from any underlying differences in approach.

The task-based rating scale that we have described in earlier chapters was developed for the VT of general practitioners. Its use in teaching depends on the teacher being able to offer alternative strategies and skills as required, and does not specify them in the scale.

The SEGUE instrument developed at Northwestern University, Chicago (Makoul 2001) is widely used in North America, and the Calgary Cambridge rating scale (Kurtz and Silverman 1996) is being used increasingly in the United Kingdom. They were both developed for undergraduates and include a mixture of tasks and skills. Instruments to assess specific aspects of communication, for example, breaking bad news (Miller *et al.* 1997), patient-centredness (Kinnersley *et al.* 1996; Mead and Bower 2000) and shared decision making (Elwyn *et al.* 2002) have been developed, but are not yet widely used in teaching or assessment.

Quality improvement

Peer review or self-assessment can be based on the same frameworks that are used in teaching. However, another approach is to collect feedback from patients using structured questionnaires (Greco *et al.* 1998). The most recent interesting example of such a tool is the measurement of 'patient enablement', carried out by asking patients to answer six questions following the consultation. The questions relate to coping, understanding, confidence, and feeling in control of one's health. When combined with the length of the consultation and an analysis of how well the patient knows the doctor, the researchers have produced a quality index of doctor's performance (Howie *et al.* 2000). The drawback of this sort of assessment is that it is not yet known what factors in the consultation influence patient enablement. This is an area for more research. When it has been done, the educational impact will increase and teachers will know much more specifically what to teach.

Regulatory assessment

In *undergraduate medical education*, many assessments have been based on consultations with standardized patients, sometimes with the patient as assessor. The scope of the scenarios offered to students is often limited. This increases the reliability and reproducibility of the assessment, and is often the only feasible approach with large student numbers. At this level it is sufficient to assess *competence*, what the student is able to do, rather than *performance*, what the doctor actually does in practice. It is essential that communication skills are assessed in undergraduate medical schools if only as a marker of their importance. However, at this stage it is disappointing that most assessments do not reflect the breadth of the communication curriculum.

In *postgraduate medical education*, the most developed assessment programme in the United Kingdom is the examination for MRCGP in the United Kingdom. The Royal College of GPs commissioned a working party in 1990 to produce a consulting skill assessment as part of their examination. One of us (PT) chaired this group, and another (DP) was part of the development group. The intention was to encourage the learning and teaching of skilful doctor–patient consulting. The examination was intended to develop the educational climate to allow more time to be spent considering communication, and for consulting competence to be seen as a high priority in the armament of future GPs. To do this a clear definition of what the candidate needed to achieve was created (Tate *et al.* 1999).

The MRCGP statement of clinical competence, derived from our task model and other expert opinion, is a comprehensive model designed for teaching and end point assessment. It uses the framework of National Vocational Qualifications, dividing the criteria into Units (tasks), Elements (strategies), and Performance Criteria (skills).

The *tasks* of the general practitioner during the consultation are defined as five units:

(1) discover the reasons for a patient's attendance;

(2) define the clinical problem(s);

(3) explain the problem(s) to the patient;

(4) address the patient's problem(s);

(5) make effective use of the consultation.

Each of these units is subdivided into *elements*. For example in unit one—discover the reasons for the patient's attendance—there are four elements:

(1) elicit the patient's account of the symptom(s) that made him/her turn to the doctor;

(2) obtain relevant items of social and occupational circumstances;

(3) explore the patient's health understanding;

(4) enquire about continuing problems.

The tasks are too broad to be reliably assessed even at this level. There follows an even more specific level called *'Performance Criteria'* (PC). Each element of the definition has one or more PC. For example, for the *unit*, 'discover the reasons for the patient's attendance' and the *element* 'elicit the patient's account of the symptoms which made him/her turn to the doctor', there are two PC: 'the doctor encourages the patient's contribution at appropriate points in the consultation', and 'the doctor responds to cues'.

The total list of PC is as follows:

1. The doctor is seen to encourage the patient's contribution at appropriate points in the consultation.

2. The doctor is seen to respond to cues that are present in the consultation.

3. The doctor elicits appropriate details sufficient to place the complaint(s) in a social and psychological context.

4. (M) The doctor takes the patient's health understanding into account.

5. The doctor obtains sufficient information for no serious condition to be missed.

6. The physical examination chosen is likely to confirm or disprove the hypotheses that could reasonably have been formed *or* is designed to address a patient's concern.

7. The doctor appears to make a clinically appropriate working diagnosis.

8. The doctor explains the diagnosis, management, and effects of treatment.

9. The content of what the doctor says and the language used is appropriate to what the patient needs.

10. (M) The doctor explains utilizing some or all of the patient's elicited beliefs.

11. (M) The doctor is seen to make an effort to confirm the patient's understanding.

12. The management plan is appropriate for the working diagnosis, reflecting a good understanding of modern accepted medical practice.

13. The doctor shares management options with the patient.

14. The doctor establishes an effective rapport with the patient.

15. The doctor prescribes appropriately.

The three criteria labelled (M) are criteria for the award of a merit. In order to clarify these definitions further, the candidates are provided with even more detailed descriptions of the requirements in a workbook.

The underlying philosophy of this assessment methodology is a demonstration of consulting ability by the assessed: the demonstration of 'can do'. This imposes the educational burden on the candidate to recognize the criteria and to demonstrate them. This is totally compatible with our educational aims in teaching and learning from the seven tasks. The burden of proof is handed to the candidate: having been told in fine detail what is required of them, they must produce a videotape that demonstrates their competence against required PC.

The candidates for this assessment should:

♦ know which competences must be demonstrated;

♦ conform to rules governing the submission of evidence;

♦ be guided by a mentor or trainer;

♦ submit the evidence when it is ready.

Videotape is used for direct observation. This places the assessment at the summit of Miller's pyramid and ensures that validity is high. The Royal College examiners consider the seven selected consultation on the videotape to be a *portfolio of competence*: a collection of effective consultations put together over a period of time.

Other groups have used standardized patients in multiple-station examinations and compared these with assessments in practice and found that the assessments in practice were more valid, and as reliable, as those in the more controlled setting (Ram *et al.* 1999).

Results of the video assessment

Over 3000 candidates have been assessed by this methodology to date. The reliability has been found to be high ($\alpha = 0.89$). The overall failure rate of the component is about 30 per cent. Of the candidates that failed, most were deemed by the examiners to have failed to demonstrate competence in two or more PC. The most commonly absent PC, in descending order, are:

(1) the doctor shares management options with the patient;

(2) the doctor elicits appropriate details to place the complaint in a social and psychological context;

(3) the doctor responds to cues;

(4) the doctor's management plan is appropriate for the working diagnosis;

(5) the doctor explains the diagnosis, management, and effects of treatment;

(6) The doctor explains in language appropriate to the patient.

The three merit criteria are deliberately intended to be 'patient-centred':

(1) the doctor takes the patient's health understanding into account;

(2) the doctor explains utilizing some or all of the patient's elicited beliefs;

(3) the doctor is seen to make an effort to confirm the patient's understanding.

Currently less than 10 per cent of candidates are demonstrating patient-centred behaviour.

UK Royal Colleges

Other UK medical Royal Colleges are including communication skill assessment as part of their professional examinations. The Royal College of Physicians included a communication skills and ethics station in their clinical examination for the first time with the following criteria:

1. Communication skills—conduct of the interview

   (a) introduces self to patient and explains role clearly;

   (b) agrees the purpose of the interview with the patient;

   (c) puts the patient at ease and establishes good rapport;

   (d) explores the patient's concerns, feelings, and expectations—demonstrates empathy, respect, and non-judgemental attitude;

   (e) prioritizes problems and redirects the interview sensitively.

2. Communication skills—exploration and problem negotiation

   (a) appropriate questioning style—generally open-ended to closed as the interview progresses;

(b) provides clear explanations (jargon free) that the patient understands;

(c) agrees a clear course of action;

(d) summarizes and checks the patient's understanding;

(e) concludes the interview appropriately.

3. Ethics and law:

(a) in relation to the clinical scenario, the candidates demonstrate knowledge of the relevant ethical and legal principles and appropriate attitudes in making decisions;

(b) knowledge of ethical principles;

(c) understanding of legal constraints applicable to the case;

(d) provides adequate reasoning as appropriate to the case.

It can be seen that the approaches of the colleges is similar and patient-centred consulting is required by all of them.

Summary

1. Assessment is an essential part of the educational process to identify needs, monitor progress, and assure satisfactory performance.

2. By assessing one's learners, we can also evaluate our effectiveness as teachers.

3. To develop reliable and valid assessments of patient-centred consulting is important in teaching, quality assessment, regulatory assessments, and research.

11 Implementation of the approach to teaching and learning

Introduction

Our original approach to learning and teaching the consultation had two principal elements. The first was a model of an effective consultation which included not only the clinical task of establishing the nature of the patient's problem and its aetiology, but also exploring the patient's ideas, concerns and expectations about the problem and its management. It also included sharing understanding, decisions, and responsibility with patients. The second was a method of teaching that was based on observing how effectively a doctor achieved the tasks in a consultation, and giving feedback that identified her strengths, and ways in which she could become more effective.

There were a number of parallels between these processes. We were describing a patient centred style of consulting in which the central purpose was to identify and to meet the patient's needs, and a similar, learner-centred style of teaching in which the learner was encouraged to identify her own strengths and weaknesses and negotiate the agenda for her teaching. We also described the consultation as part of a cycle of care in which patients' understanding and ability to manage their own health were enhanced at each consultation. Similarly, the central purpose of our teaching is to help our learners understand their own consultation style and the ways in which they could develop and become more effective.

In earlier chapters in this book we have described these approaches, and the ways in which our ideas have developed in the light of experience. In this chapter we will discuss how clinical practice and teaching are changing, and some of the challenges we continue to face.

Diffusion of innovations

Patient-centred consulting and learner-centred teaching were both innovations that we, amongst many others, wished to see implemented in practice. Producing change is a complex and difficult process. One description of this process that we have found very helpful is the 'Diffusion of Innovations' model by Everett Rogers (1995). This defines diffusion as the process by which an innovation is communicated through certain channels over time and becomes adopted by the members of a social system. The factors that can influence the rate at which a new practice is adopted, or whether it is adopted at all, include the nature of the innovation itself, the relationship between it's proponents and potential adopters, the characteristics of the adopters themselves, and the social system within which diffusion takes place.

Introduction of learner-centred communication skills teaching

1. The nature of the innovation

The characteristics of an innovation that determine its rate of adoption are its:

◆ relative advantage over existing practice

◆ compatibility with existing values and practice

◆ complexity (difficulty to understand and use)

◆ 'trialability' (the degree to which it can be tried on a limited basis)

◆ observability (visibility to others).

There is no question that general practice trainers believed that our approach to teaching fulfilled these requirements. The importance of the doctor–patient relationship as the core of general practice was part of the shared values of GP teachers and being patient- and learner-centred felt right. Structured methods of observation and feedback were preferred to the critical comments that often came from the teacher comparing the learner with the teacher herself! Though the practice and teaching of patient-centred consulting is a complex and difficult task, our approach divided it into its component parts. Reducing the degree of complexity and threat, allowing trainers to try out the approach in a protected environment, and giving them the opportunity to observe others doing so, were also appreciated in the trainers' workshops described earlier.

2. The proponents and adopters

Our approach was developed over a number of years. The process involved active debate and development amongst the authors, and testing out of the acceptability and feasibility of these ideas by presenting them to a series of teachers' courses. This was a very important and valuable part of the process, as we were able to incorporate a much wider range of views than our own, albeit those of trainers alone, and our eventual publication reflected this consensus. However, once the ideas were crystallized and published, there was a danger that they could become an orthodoxy.

As well as improving the product, this method of development reduced the distance between the innovators and the adopters, and created a degree of ownership of the ideas amongst a body of credible opinion leaders in their local trainers' groups who acted as our advocates. Trainers, particularly those who go on new courses, are likely to be early adopters of new ideas, while late adopters are more likely to be isolated and have less positive attitudes to, and experience of, change.

3. The social system

As well as the relatively informal networks of courses and workshops, trainers are also part of a structured accreditation and re-accreditation system of training practice assessments. Once the majority of trainers had adopted any innovation it was possible to include encouragement or even sanctions to ensure that 'laggards' also implemented our approach (Rogers' word, not ours!). Thus, over the years, trainers have been asked to show at least one of their own consultations to the visiting assessors, and use it to demonstrate teaching.

Whilst the notion of sanctions may seem unduly authoritarian, Rogers' work implies that there is a natural influence sequence that innovators need to understand and use. The process moves through co-development of ideas, and involvement, through the provision of proof, to eventual compulsion—but only to influence the last few members of a group when the rest are on board and where consistency is required. The introduction of the observation of recorded consultations as a method of assessment in the Examination of the Royal College of General Practitioners with criteria derived from our tasks, is a mark of the general acceptance of our work, and a very powerful encouragement to all teachers and learners to ensure that teaching takes place.

We know that communication skills teaching has been widely adopted in vocational training (VT) for general practice in the United Kingdom, and in many other countries. In 1995 two of us (TS and PH) sent a questionnaire to all the trainers, course organisers and advisors in the Oxford region seeking their views, use of, and blocks to consultation teaching. About 97 per cent of trainers in the region had easy access to a video camera and over 60 per cent of trainees had their consultations reviewed four times a year or more. The blocks to effective teaching, if any, were time rather than lack of skill or lack of belief in the need for consultation skills teaching. A similar survey in the West Midlands (Field 1995) found that 93 per cent of trainers used video recording for teaching and that our framework was the commonest used assessment tool. There are now courses for communication skills teachers in many parts of the United Kingdom, and some of these have drawn on approaches developed in North America (Bird *et al.* 1993).

The evidence shows that our approach seems to have influenced teaching. The evidence that there has been a comparable change in clinical practice is much less convincing. The research study that we conducted based on recorded consultations by volunteer general practitioners, a proportion of whom were our trainers, have shown great variation in the degree to which our tasks were achieved in those consultations (Makoul *et al.* 1995). John Howie, with

170 general practitioners who were again volunteers, showed a wide variation in the quality of their consultations as measured by an index based on consultation length, patient enablement and continuity of care (Howie 1999). Stevenson *et al.* (2000) found very little shared decision-making in their sample of 62 consultations. In this, as in many other areas, the challenge remains to bridge the gap between theory and evidence on the one hand and practice on the other.

4. The innovation

The difficulty was, and remains, that a patient-centred approach to consulting can be seen as less advantageous and more risky than more traditional styles learned at medical school. Exploring the patient's ideas and concerns can be seen as more time consuming, and 'opening a can of worms'. Given the opportunity, patients may express views that are assertive or critical. Patients vary widely in their desire for, and their expectation to be involved in, decisions about their care, and initially can be more concerned if asked to be involved. Further, there a small but widely quoted studies purported to show that patients prefer an authoritative style of doctoring (Savage and Armstrong 1990) and that clumsy attempts at being patient-centred, such as 'What do you think is wrong with you?', may be felt to undermine the doctor's authority. However more recent and rigorous studies have demonstrated the patients' preference for a patient centred approach (Little *et al.* 2001).

This all means that the experience of the doctor who is starting to make changes in his style may not be immediately rewarding. Byrne and Long (1976) pointed out that a closed, doctor-centred style of consulting can be self-perpetuating, and that 'once a doctor develops their style, there is a danger that it becomes a prison within which they are forced to work'.

Evidence that supports patient-centred clinical methods has been systematically reviewed earlier. It is derived from many disciplines and countries, but there are few studies in UK general practice. Those that have been done have failed to show positive effects of patient-centred care on clinical outcomes (Kinmonth *et al.* 1998; Pill *et al.* 1998; Kinnersley *et al.* 1999).

5. The proponents

Innovators who argue for change are social deviants, and are less credible than opinion leaders amongst the adopters of the change. This is exacerbated if the innovators come from outside, either from 'academic practice' or from other disciplines. These perceptions can create a gulf between teachers and practising doctors that is difficult to bridge, in spite of protests that the teachers are practising doctors as well.

The investment in Vocational Training for General Practice in the United Kingdom was based on the belief that improving the knowledge and skills of new entrants to the profession will produce changes that are taken up by its more senior members. This may have worked for organizational developments such as audit, but it is a very weak strategy for achieving change in the consulting style of established doctors. Teaching the teachers on the other hand, ostensibly about teaching but also about practice, has been much more effective as they tend to be opinion leaders in their practices. However this again tends to widen the gulf between those involved in teaching and those who are not.

6. The adopters

There are two groups of adopters with whom we are concerned. The first is the doctors emerging from undergraduate education and postgraduate training for general practice. The extent to which they are, or are not, able to display patient-centred consulting behaviours in the Membership of the Royal College of General Practitioners (MRCGP) examination has been discussed earlier. The overall impression of the persistence of doctor-centred behaviours may just be because our teaching is ineffective, but it may indicate problems in their previous training and the system within which they have been acquiring their consulting habits.

The selection process for medical school with its emphasis on performance in examinations and interviews will tend to select scientific doers and talkers rather than reflective listeners. The role models, and particularly the process of clinical teaching, encourages the 'Taking' of histories and the making of clinical diagnoses. The 'clinical material' from which the students learn usually involves patients with serious conditions, so the emphasis is on diagnosis and treatment delivered by doctors and nurses, rather than longer-term care with patient and carer involvement. The work of a junior hospital doctor—its time pressures, the amount of disease and distress, and common lack of personal support—means that many young doctors develop survival strategies which include a closed, doctor-centred style of consulting. Vocational training for general practice therefore becomes a remedial exercise in which communication skills teaching is only a part.

The second group of doctors who we hope will adopt the innovation of patient-centred consulting is established practitioners: a widely varied group of doctors with whom generalizations are dangerous. As has already been mentioned any study of consultation behaviours is necessarily based on volunteers, but those that have been carried out on substantial samples of British general practitioners do not show evidence of a large increase in patient-centred behaviours over this time. This may reflect limitations in the approach, the failure of the proponents to engage with established doctors and their continued education, and the effects of the system within which the doctors work.

In our first book there was no chapter called 'Understanding the doctor' and it is fair to say that attempts to change clinical practice have frequently failed to take this understanding into account. While we recognize how difficult it is to change patients' behaviour we do not often consider doctors' 'Readiness to change' or 'Health Beliefs'.

In the United Kingdom those doctors who are responsible for *continuing professional development (CPD)* have on the whole been less well paid, trained, and supported than those involved in Vocational Training. They are often dependent on the pharmaceutical industry for financial support for their meetings, which means that if communication is discussed at all it is in the context of achieving compliance with medication. Additionally, there has been no system of performance review or support that involves all doctors, particularly one that looks at their communication with patients, although Clinical Governance may provide this in the future. Clinical Governance is starting in many places with a narrow view of quality of care but some innovative schemes are including patient assessments of quality and the inclusion of the assessments of the quality of the consultations.

The system

There is a danger in 'blaming the system' for any difficulties as it absolves the individuals from accepting personal responsibility and suggests that change is impossible. However, there is a growing recognition that quality of health care depends as much on the system as on the professionals working within it, and that ignoring failures in the system risks inappropriate 'victim blaming'. Some features of the UK healthcare system have to be recognized.

Primary care consultations tend to be short. In the United Kingdom the average length is about eight minutes and it is frequently argued that this limits the range of issues that can be explored, the amount of information that can be given and the amount that patients can be involved in choices in the consultation. The available evidence supports this view (Freeman *et al.* 2002).

There is a complex interaction between *accessibility* (how soon a patient has to wait to see a doctor), *continuity* (whether they see the same doctor), and the *length of consultations*, all operating within the overall *availability of resources*. Many health care systems, including British general practice, set a limit on the number and cost of doctors, so time becomes the resource that is rationed or managed above all. Systems which provide greater accessibility may do this at the cost of less continuity or shorter consultations. Patients who have longer consultations with a doctor that they know, may be more enabled to manage their own problems and need fewer consultations over time, but may wait longer for them.

The individual doctor is usually unable to alter the overall resources, but has some control over the length, and more control over the content, of their consultations. The pressures on time, both in hospital and in general practice partnerships, is immense and is frequently offered as the principal reason why change is so difficult to achieve.

Most health care systems have greater, or at least more immediate, rewards for quantity than quality of care. These range from approval from colleagues for 'getting through' more patients, to financial rewards for larger lists or more patient contacts. Even though the RCGP proposals to assess doctors' performance in practice, (*'What Sort of Doctor?'* 1985), included the assessment of the ability to communicate, this has not been taken up widely in the profession, with the exception of teachers in general practice. Quality measures tend to measure the measurable, not necessarily what is important.

Achieving change in the consulting room requires change not just in the individuals present, but also in the systems that support them. It is more difficult to be patient-centred in the consulting room in the absence of a *patient-centred environment*, including the physical surroundings, the attitudes of reception staff, waiting times and the availability of information. In many parts of the National Health Service these are woefully lacking.

Possible solutions

It is possible to use the analysis provided by the Diffusion of Innovations model to consider how the uptake of patient-centred consulting in practice could be enhanced.

The innovation

The *presentation and packaging* of our approach could have been improved earlier to make it clearer and more memorable. For this reason, we have now made the key issues in the task list to read as follows:

◆ understand the problem

◆ understand the patient

◆ share understanding

◆ share decisions and responsibility

◆ maintain the relationship

... and do all this within the allocated time.

This also fits onto five fingers!

Some *simple rules* for achieving the tasks could be devised that would make the approach more memorable. For example:

1. Before considering a prescription always ask 'Do you want me to give you something for this?'

2. Before a prescription for an antibiotic ask 'What do you feel about taking/ giving your child an antibiotic?'

3. Before giving your diagnosis ask 'What thoughts have been running through your mind?'

4. Before embarking on an explanation ask 'What do you understand about...?

These questions may appear simplistic but they have the advantage of making the message practical, and they will also obtain immediate feedback from the patient that will reinforce the message. They may also lead to fewer prescriptions and shorter explanations. These questions are the demonstration of the underlying single message that would help the doctor practice patient-centred medicine, develop a real curiosity; a curiosity about the patient's condition and a curiosity about the patient themselves.

As well as immediate feedback doctors need *more convincing evidence* that patient-centred consulting has the longer-term advantages that are claimed for it. Controlled trials are very difficult to conduct in this field because changing consultation styles is so difficult to achieve, but studies do need to be done that demonstrate that more enabling consultations lead to better health and to more appropriate utilization of heath services.

The proponents

The most effective change agents within a system are the local opinion leaders. In hospitals *junior hospital doctors* are the role models for medical students, and more time and resources need to be provided firstly to understand the pressures that they are under, and then to train and support them to consult in a more patient-centred way.

Senior hospital doctors can also lead opinion by making the importance of patient centred consulting more explicit. If every medical student and junior hospital doctor knew that when they presented a patient they would be asked not just for a chronological account of their symptoms but also:

1. What is this patient most concerned about?
2. What does the patient understand about his problem?
3. What would the patient like us to do for him?

They would learn the importance of the patient's perspective very quickly.

Postgraduate tutors have a more difficult job trying to achieve change in established practice, whether in hospital or general practice, than those involved in training the students. If they are to tackle established doctors' consulting styles then they will need significant training and continued support.

The most powerful and persuasive voices that argue for more partnership with patients and shared decision-making are *patients* themselves, and those that seek to represent them. Patients are becoming better informed and have higher expectations of their doctors. Patients now expect to be put at the centre of the health system, and will be content with nothing less (Coulter 2002).

We need a dialogue with patients and patient groups that helps them achieve the balance between legitimate criticism and constructive support. Above all we need a partnership with our patients to achieve some of the necessary changes in the health care system itself. This requires doctors both to make the case for, and be willing to deliver, personal and continuing care in partnership with their patients, so that it is experienced and appreciated by them.

All these proponents need the *research evidence* to support them. Controlled trials are difficult because they require interventions that demonstrably change the consulting style of the doctor, and they can feel contrived in this context. Nevertheless, we still need high quality studies, conducted in comparable settings to those in which the potential adopters work, that demonstrate that patient-centred consulting really makes a difference to outcomes for patients.

The adopters

We need to remember the principles of *adult learning and learner-centred teaching* when we approach our colleagues, and not resort to exhortation if things do not change as rapidly as we would wish. We also need to be mindful that Maslow's hierarchy of needs starts with safety, belonging and affection before self-actualization can be achieved. Patient-centred consulting can be deeply rewarding once the acquired defence mechanisms are abandoned. We have talked about creating *safe and supportive environments* to allow experimentation and change on our courses. We need to be able to do the same in clinical practice.

The system

We need a *consistent message* that effective communication between the institutions and professionals on the one hand and the public and patients on the other is the central determinant of the quality of any health care system. Communicating this message within any organization will only be effective if the words, the actions and the allocation of resources and rewards are all consistent. The words need to come from patients and their organizations, professionals and their Colleges, and government and their managers. The actions are largely about changes in professional attitudes and practice, and about all stages of professional education. The resources, particularly the resources to allow professionals adequate time with their patients, come via governments in state funded systems, and directly from patients in others. The challenge is to be able to match capacity with demand, and to make both realistic.

Together with patients we need to be able to set targets for the quality of our communication, and include them in our *quality measures* and in international comparisons of health care systems. Clinical guidelines and policies need to be developed in partnership with patients, and need to state clearly that patients' preferences and values should be taken into account in shared decision making about their care.

In the United Kingdom we need to take the government at its word that it intends to provide a 'First Class Service' and work with them to do so, but also challenge the primacy of access as a quality target to the exclusion of consultation length or continuity of care. Clinical Governance is 'A framework through which NHS organizations are accountable for continuously improving the quality of their services and safeguarding high standards of care by creating an environment in which excellence in clinical care will flourish' (NHS 1998). We need to build-in effective communication as a central part of this framework. It is to be expected that audits and reviews will tend to measure the measurable. We therefore need to develop robust measures of communication and of patient-centred outcomes of care such as informed choice. Reward systems should be based on these measures.

Patient-centred consulting and partnerships between patients, professionals, and the government should be rewarding for us all.

References

Arborelius, E. and Bremberg, S. (1992), 'What can doctors do to achieve a successful consultation? Videotaped interviews analysed by the "consultation map" method', *Fam. Pract.*, **9**(1), 61–6.

Association of American Medical Colleges (1998), *Learning objectives for medical student education. Guidelines for medical schools*, Association of American Medical Colleges, Washington DC.

Balint, M. (1957), *The doctor, his patient and the illness*, Churchill Livingstone, Edinburgh.

Bandura, A. (1977), 'Self-efficacy: toward a unifying theory of behavioral change', *Psychol. Rev.*, **84**(2), 191–215.

Barker, D. J., Forsen, T., Uutela, A., Osmond, C., and Eriksson, J. G. (2001), 'Size at birth and resilience to effects of poor living conditions in adult life: longitudinal study', *BMJ*, **323**(7324), 1273–6.

Bass, M. J., Buck, C., Turner, L., Dickie, G., Pratt, G., and Robinson, H. C. (1986), 'The physician's actions and the outcome of illness in family practice', *J. Fam. Pract.*, **23**(1), 43–7.

Beauchamp, T. L. and Childress, J. F. (1979), *Principles of biomedical ethics*, Oxford University Press, New York.

Becker, M. H. (1974), 'The health belief model and sick role behaviour', *Health Educ. Monogr.*, (2), 409–19.

Becker, M. H. (1982), *Social science perspectives on primary care*, paper presented at Social Science and Primary Care Conference, University of Oxford.

Becker, M. H. and Maiman, L. A. (1975), 'Sociobehavioral determinants of compliance with health and medical care recommendations', *Med. Care*, **13**(1), 10–24.

Beckman, H. B. and Frankel, R. M. (1984), 'The effect of physician behavior on the collection of data', *Ann. Intern. Med.*, **101**(5), 692–6.

Beckman, H. B., Kaplan, S. H., and Frankel, R. (1989), 'Outcome-based research on doctor–patient communication: a review', in: M. Stewart & D. Roter (eds), *Communicating with medical patients*, Sage Publications, Newbury Park, CA.

Beckman, H. B., Markakis, K. M., Suchman, A. L., and Frankel, R. M. (1994), 'The doctor–patient relationship and malpractice. Lessons from plaintiff depositions', *Arch. Intern. Med.*, **154**(12), 1365–70.

Bensing, J. (2000), 'Bridging the gap. The separate worlds of evidence-based medicine and patient-centered medicine', *Patient Educ. Couns.*, **39**(1), 17–25.

Bird, J., Hall, A., Maguire, P., and Heavy, A. (1993), 'Workshops for consultants on the teaching of clinical communication skills', *Med. Educ.*, **27**(2), 181–5.

Black, D. (1980), *Inequalities in Health*, Department of Health and Social Security, London.

Boreham, P. and Gibson, D. (1978), 'The informative process in private medical consultations: a preliminary investigation', *Soc. Sci. Med.*, **12**(5A), 409–16.

Britten, N. and Ukoumunne, O. (1997), 'The influence of patients' hopes of receiving a prescription on doctors' perceptions and the decision to prescribe: a questionnaire survey', *BMJ*, **315**(7121), 1506–10.

Britten, N., Stevenson, F. A., Barry, C. A., Barber, N., and Bradley, C. P. (2000), 'Misunderstandings in prescribing decisions in general practice: qualitative study', *BMJ*, **320**(7233), 484–8.

Brody, D. S., Miller, S. M., Lerman, C. E., Smith, D. G., and Caputo, G. C. (1989), 'Patient perception of involvement in medical care: relationship to illness attitudes and outcomes', *J. Gen. Intern. Med.*, **4**(6), 506–11.

Butler, C. C. and Evans, M. (1999), 'The "heartsink" patient revisited. The Welsh Philosophy and General Practice discussion Group', *Br. J. Gen. Pract.*, **49**(440), 230–3.

Butler, C. C., Rollnick, S., and Stott, N. (1996), 'The practitioner, the patient and resistance to change: recent ideas on compliance', *CMAJ*, **154**(9), 1357–62.

Byrne, P. and Long, B. (1976), *Doctors talking to patients*, HMSO, London.

Charles, C., Gafni, A., and Whelan, T. (1997), 'Shared decision-making in the medical encounter: what does it mean? (or it takes at least two to tango)', *Soc. Sci. Med.*, **44**(5), 681–92.

Charles, C., Whelan, T., and Gafni, A. (1999), 'What do we mean by partnership in making decisions about treatment?', *BMJ*, **319**(7212), 780–2.

Cohen-Cole, S. A. (1991), *The medical interview: the three-function approach*, Mosby Year Book, St Louis.

Coulter, A., Peto, V., and Doll, H. (1994), 'Patients' preferences and general practitioners' decisions in the treatment of menstrual disorders', *Fam. Pract.*, **11**(1), 67–74.

Coulter, A. (1997), 'Partnerships with patients: The pros and cons of shared clinical decision-making', *J. Health Services Res. Policy*, **2**, 112–21.

Coulter, A., Entwistle, V., and Gilbert, D. (1999), 'Sharing decisions with patients: is the information good enough?', *BMJ*, **318**(7179), 318–22.

Coulter, A. (2002), 'After Bristol: putting patients at the centre', *BMJ*, **324**(7338), 648–51.

Crawford, R. (1984), 'A cultural account of "health" control, release and the social body', in J. B. McKinlay (ed.), *Issues in the political economy of health care*, Tavistock, New York.

Dixon, D. M., Sweeney, K. G., and Gray, D. J. (1999), 'The physician healer: ancient magic or modern science?', *Br. J. Gen. Pract.*, **49**(441), 309–12.

Edwards, A., Elwyn, G., and Mulley, A. (2002), 'Explaining risks: turning numerical data into meaningful pictures', *BMJ*, **324**(7341), 827–30.

Elwyn, G., Edwards, A., Gwyn, R., and Grol, R. (1999), 'Towards a feasible model for shared decision making: focus group study with general practice registrars', *BMJ*, **319**(7212), 753–6.

Elwyn, G., Edwards, A., and Kinnersley, P. (1999), 'Shared decision-making in primary care: the neglected second half of the consultation', *Br. J. Gen. Pract.*, **49**(443), 477–82.

Elwyn, G., Edwards, A., Wensing, M., Atwell, C., Hood, K., and Grol, R. (2002), 'Fleeting glimpses: measuring shared decision making in primary care using the OPTION instrument', *Medical Decision Making*, in Press.

Fallowfield, L. J., Hall, A., Maguire, G. P., and Baum, M. (1990), 'Psychological outcomes of different treatment policies in women with early breast cancer outside a clinical trial [see comments]', *BMJ*, **301**(6752), 575–80.

Field, S. (1995), 'The use of video recording in general practice: a survey of trainers in the West Midlands region', *Educ. General Practice*, **6**, 49–58.

Fitton, F. and Acheson, H. W. (1979), *The doctor patient relationship*, HMSO, London.

Fitzpatrick, R. M., Hopkins, A. P., and Harvard Watts, O. (1983), 'Social dimensions of healing: a longitudinal study of outcomes of medical management of headaches', *Soc. Sci. Med.*, **17**(8), 501–10.

Ford, S., Fallowfield, L., and Lewis, S. (1996), 'Doctor–patient interactions in oncology', *Soc. Sci. Med.*, **42**(11), 1511–19.

Freeman, G. K., Horder, J. P., Howie, J. G., Hungin, A. P., Hill, A. P., Shah, N. C., and Wilson, A. (2002), 'Evolving general practice consultation in Britain: issues of length and context', *BMJ*, **324**(7342), 880–82.

Fugelli, P. (2001), 'James Mackenzie Lecture. Trust—in general practice', *Br. J. Gen. Pract.*, **51**(468), 575–9.

General Medical Council (1993), *Tomorrow's doctors. Recommendations on undergraduate medical education*, General Medical Council, London.

General Medical Council (1998), *Good medical practice*, General Medical Council, London.

Gray, D. P. (1998), 'Forty-seven minutes a year for the patient', *Br. J. Gen. Pract.*, **48**(437), 1816–17.

Greco, M., Francis, W., Buckley, J., Brownlea, A., and McGovern, J. (1998), 'Real-patient evaluation of communication skills teaching for GP registrars', *Fam. Pract.*, **15**(1), 51–7.

Greenfield, S., Kaplan, S., and Ware, J. E. Jr. (1985), 'Expanding patient involvement in care. Effects on patient outcomes', *Ann. Intern. Med.*, **102**(4), 520–8.

Greenhaugh, T. and Hurwitz, B. (1998), *Narrative Based Medicine: dialogue and discourse in clinical practice*, British Medical Journal, London.

Grol, R. (ed.) (1989), *To heal or to harm. The prevention of somatic fixation in general practice*, RCGP, London.

Hall, J. A., Roter, D. L., and Katz, N. R. (1988), 'Meta-analysis of correlates of provider behavior in medical encounters', *Med. Care*, **26**(7), 657–75.

Hannay, D. R. (1979), *The symptom iceberg*, Routledge and Kegan Paul, London.

Hargie, O., Dickson, D., Boohan, M., and Hughes, K. (1998), 'A survey of communication skills training in UK Schools of Medicine: Present practices and prospective proposals', *Med. Educ.*, **32**(1), 25–34.

Havelock, P., Hasler, J., Flew, R., McIntyre, D., Schofield, T., and Toby, J. (1995), *Professional education for general practice,* Oxford University Press, Oxford.

Haynes, R. B., McKibbon, K. A., and Kanani, R. (1996), 'Systematic review of randomised trials of interventions to assist patients to follow prescriptions for medications', *Lancet*, **348**(9024), 383–6.

Hays, R. (1990), 'Measuring consultation process', *Postgrad. Ed. Gen. Prac.*, **1**, 139–47.

Heath, I. (1995), *The mystery of general practice*, Nuffield Trust, London.

Herxheimer, A., McPherson, A., Miller, R., Shepperd, S., Yaphe, J., and Ziebland, S. (2000), 'Database of patients' experiences (DIPEx): a multi-media approach to sharing experiences and information', *Lancet*, **355**(9214), 1540–3.

Hjortdahl, P. and Laerum, E. (1992), 'Continuity of care in general practice: effect on patient satisfaction', *BMJ*, **304**(6837), 1287–90.

Howie, J. G., Heaney, D. J., and Maxwell, M. (1997), 'Measuring quality in general practice. Pilot study of a needs, process and outcome measure', *Occas. Pap. R. Coll. Gen. Pract.* 75, i–xii, 1–32.

Howie, J. G., Heaney, D. J., Maxwell, M., and Walker, J. J. (1998), 'A comparison of a Patient Enablement Instrument (PEI) against two established satisfaction scales as an outcome measure of primary care consultations', *Fam. Pract.*, **15**(2), 165–71.

Howie, J. G., Heaney, D. J., Maxwell, M., Walker, J. J., Freeman, G. K., and Rai, H. (1999), 'Quality at general practice consultations: cross sectional survey', *BMJ*, **319**(7212), 738–43.

Howie, J. G., Heaney, D. J., Maxwell, M., Walker, J. J., and Freeman, G. K. (2000), 'Developing a "consultation quality index" (CQI) for use in general practice', *Fam. Pract.*, **17**(6), 455–61.

Illich, I. (1976), *Limits to Medicine. Medical Nemesis: The Expropriation of Health*, Marion Boyars, London.

Kagan, N., Schauble, P., Resnikoff, A., Danish, S. J., and Krathwohl, D. R. (1969), 'Interpersonal process recall', *J. Nerv. Ment. Dis.*, **148**(4), 365–74.

Kai, J. (1996), 'What worries parents when their preschool children are acutely ill, and why: a qualitative study', *BMJ*, **313**(7063), 983–6.

Kaplan, S. H., Greenfield, S., and Ware, J. E. Jr. (1989), 'Assessing the effects of physician–patient interactions on the outcomes of chronic disease', *Med. Care*, **27**(3 Suppl), S110–27.

Kearley, K. E., Freeman, G. K., and Heath, A. (2001), 'An exploration of the value of the personal doctor–patient relationship in general practice', *Br. J. Gen. Pract.*, **51**(470), 712–18.

King, J. (1999), 'Giving Feedback', *BMJ*, **318**, 2.

Kinmonth, A. L., Woodcock, A., Griffin, S., Spiegal, N., and Campbell, M. J. (1998), 'Randomised controlled trial of patient centred care of diabetes in general practice: impact on current wellbeing and future disease risk. The Diabetes Care From Diagnosis Research Team', *BMJ*, **317**(7167), 1202–8.

Kinnersley, P., Stott, N., Peters, T., Harvey, I., and Hackett, P. (1996), 'A comparison of methods for measuring patient satisfaction with consultations in primary care', *Fam. Pract.*, **13**(1), 41–51.

Kinnersley, P., Stott, N., Peters, T. J., and Harvey, I. (1999), 'The patient-centredness of consultations and outcome in primary care', *Br. J. Gen. Pract.*, **49**(446), 711–16.

Kolb, D. (1984), *Experiential learning: Experience as a source of learning and development*, Prentice Hall, Englewood Cliffs.

Kurtz, S., Silverman, J., and Draper, J. (1998), *Teaching and learning communication skills in medicine*, Radcliffe Medical Press, Abingdon.

Kurtz, S. M. and Silverman, J. D. (1996), 'The Calgary-Cambridge Referenced Observation Guides: an aid to defining the curriculum and organizing the teaching in communication training programmes', *Med. Educ.*, **30**(2), 83–9.

Lassen, L. C. (1991), 'Connections between the quality of consultations and patient compliance in general practice', *Fam. Pract.*, **8**(2), 154–60.

Levenstein, J. H., McCracken, E. C., McWhinney, I. R., Stewart, M. A., and Brown, J. B. (1986), 'The patient-centred clinical method. 1. A model for the doctor–patient interaction in family medicine', *Fam. Pract.*, **3**(1), 24–30.

Leventhal, H. and Cameron, L. (1987), 'Behavioural theories and the problem of compliance', *Patient Edu. Couns.*, **10**, 117–38.

Ley, P. (1979), 'Memory for medical information', *Br. J. Soc. Clin. Psychol.*, **18**, 245–56.

Ley, P. (1988), *Communicating with patients: improving communication, satisfaction and compliance*, Chapman and Hall, London.

Lipkin, M. Jr., Quill, T. E., and Napodano, R. J. (1984), 'The medical interview: a core curriculum for residencies in internal medicine', *Ann. Intern. Med.*, **100**(2), 277–84.

Little, P., Everitt, H., Williamson, I., Warner, G., Moore, M., Gould, C., Ferrier, K., and Payne, S. (2001), 'Preferences of patients for patient centred approach to consultation in primary care: observational study', *BMJ*, **322**(7284), 468–72.

Little, P., Everitt, H., Williamson, I., Warner, G., Moore, M., Gould, C., Ferrier, K., and Payne, S. (2001), 'Observational study of effect of patient centredness and positive approach on outcomes of general practice consultations', *BMJ*, **323**(7318), 908–11.

Makoul, G., Arntson, P., and Schofield, T. (1995), 'Health promotion in primary care: physician–patient communication and decision making about prescription medications', *Soc. Sci. Med.*, **41**(9), 1241–54.

Makoul, G. and Schofield, T. (1999), 'Communication teaching and assessment in medical education: an international consensus statement', *Patient Edu. Coun.*, **137**, 191–5.

Makoul, G. (2001), 'The SEGUE Framework for teaching and assessing communication skills', *Patient. Educ. Couns*, **45**(1), 23–34.

Marinker, M. (1996), 'Sense and Sensibility', in Marinker, M. (ed.), *Sense and sensibility in health care*, BMJ Books, London.

Marmot, M. G., Bosma, H., Hemingway, H., Brunner, E., and Stansfeld, S. (1997), 'Contribution of job control and other risk factors to social variations in coronary heart disease incidence', *Lancet*, **350**(9073), 235–39.

Maslow, A. (1970), *Motivation and personality*, Harper and Row, New York.

Mathers, N., Jones, N., and Hannay, D. (1995), 'Heartsink patients: a study of their general practitioners', *Br. J. Gen. Pract.*, **45**(395), 293–6.

McKeowan, T. (1979), *The role of medicine: dream, mirage or nemesis?* Blackwell, Oxford.

McKinstry, B. (2000), 'Do patients wish to be involved in decision making in the consultation? A cross sectional survey with video vignettes', *BMJ*, **321**(7265), 867–71.

McWhinney, I. (1995), 'Why we need a new clinical method', in *Patient-centered medicine: transforming the clinical method*, M. Stewart *et al.*, (eds), Sage, Thousand Oaks.

Mead, N. and Bower, P. (2000), 'Patient-centredness: a conceptual framework and review of the empirical literature', *Soc. Sci. Med.*, **51**(7), 1087–110.

Mead, N. and Bower, P. (2000), 'Measuring patient-centredness: a comparison of three observation-based instruments', *Patient Educ. Couns*, **39**(1), 71–80.

Metcalfe, D. (1999), 'Medical Schools: a poor preparation for general practice', in Moreton, P. (ed.), *The very stuff of general practice*, Radcliffe Medical Press, Abingdon.

Mezirow, D. (1981), 'A critical theory of adult learning and education', *Adult Education*, **32**, 3–24.

Miller, G. E. (1990), 'The assessment of clinical skills/competence/ performance', *Acad. Med.*, **65**(9 Suppl), S63–7.

Miller, S. J., Hope, T., and Talbot, D. C. (1999), 'The development of a structured rating schedule (the BAS) to assess skills in breaking bad news', *Br. J. Cancer*, **80**(5–6), 792–800.

Miller, W. R. (1983), 'Motivational interviewing with problem drinkers', *Behav. Psycho.*, **11**(2), 147–72.

Neighbour, R. (1987), *The inner consultation: how to develop an effective and intuitive consulting style*, Kluwer Academic Publisher, Lancaster.

Novack, D. H. (1987), 'Therapeutic aspects of the clinical encounter', *J. Gen. Intern. Med.*, **2**(5), 346–55.

O'Connor, A. M., Rostom, A., Fiset, V., Tetroe, J., Entwistle, V., Llewellyn-Thomas, H., Holmes-Rovner, M., Barry, M., and Jones, J. (1999), 'Decision aids for patients facing health treatment or screening decisions: systematic review', *BMJ*, **319**(7212), 731–4.

O'Dowd, T. C. (1988), 'Five years of heartsink patients in general practice', *BMJ*, **297**(6647), 528–30.

Parsons, T. (1951), *The social system*, Free Press, New York.

Pendleton, D. (1981), *Doctor–patient communication*, D. Phil., University of Oxford.

Pendleton, D. (1983), 'Doctor–patient communication: a review', in D. Pendleton and J. Hasler (eds), *Doctor–patient communication*, Academic Press, London.

Pendleton, D., Schofield, T., Tate, P., and Havelock, P. (1984), *The consultation: an approach to learning and teaching*, Oxford university Press, Oxford.

Pill, R., Stott, N. C., Rollnick, S. R., and Rees, M. (1998), 'A randomized controlled trial of an intervention designed to improve the care given in general practice to Type II diabetic patients: patient outcomes and professional ability to change behaviour', *Fam. Pract.*, **15**(3), 229–35.

Prochaska, J. O. and DiClemente, C. C. (1986), 'Toward a comprehensive model of change', in R. Miller and N. Heather (eds), *Treating Addictive Behaviors*, Plenum Press, New York.

Ram, P., van, d. V, Rethans, J. J., Grol, R., and Aretz, K. (1999), 'Assessment of practicing family physicians: comparison of observation in a multiple-station examination using standardized patients with observation of consultations in daily practice', *Acad. Med.*, **74**(1), 62–9.

Ram, P., Grol, R., Rethans, J. J., Schouten, B., van, d. V, and Kester, A. (1999), 'Assessment of general practitioners by video observation of communicative and medical performance in daily practice: issues of validity, reliability and feasibility', *Med. Educ.*, **33**(6), 447–54.

Rethans, J. J. and Saebu, L. (1997), 'Do general practitioners act consistently in real practice when they meet the same patient twice? Examination of intradoctor variation using standardised (simulated) patients', *BMJ*, **314**(7088), 1170–3.

Ridsdale, L., Morgan, M., and Morris, R. (1992), 'Doctors' interviewing technique and its response to different booking time', *Fam. Pract.*, **9**(1), 57–60.

Rogers, E. (1983), *Diffusion of innovations*, The Free Press, New York.

Rogers, E. (1995), *Diffusion of innovations*, 4th edition, Free Press, New York.

Rogers, C. R. (1951), *Client-centered therapy*, Houghton Mifflin, Boston.

Roter, D. L., Hall, J. A., and Katz, N. R. (1988), 'Patient–physician communication: A descriptive summary of the literature', *Patient. Educ. Couns*, **12**(2), 99–119.

Roter, D. L. and Hall, J. A. (1989), 'Studies of doctor–patient interaction', *Annu. Rev. Public Health*, **10**, 163–80.

Roter, D. L., Stewart, M., Putnam, S. M., Lipkin, M. Jr., Stiles, W., and Inui, T. S. (1997), 'Communication patterns of primary care physicians', *JAMA*, **277**(4), 350–6.

Rotter (1966), 'Generalised expectancies for internal vs. external control of reinforcement', *Psychol. Mono.*, **80**.

Royal College of Practitioners (1985), *What sort of doctor?: Assessing quality of care in general practice*, Royal College of General Practitioners, London, 23.

Royal Pharmaceutical Society (1996), *Partnership in medicine taking: a consultative document*, RPSGB, London.

Salinsky, J. and Sackin, P. (2000), *What are you feeling Doctor? Identifying and avoiding defensive patterns in the consultation*, Radcliffe Medical Press, Abingdon.

Savage, R. and Armstrong, D. (1990), 'Effect of a general practitioner's consulting style on patients' satisfaction: a controlled study [published erratum appears in *BMJ* (1990) Dec 8; **301**(6764),1316] [see comments]', *BMJ*, **301**(6758), 968–70.

Schwenk, T. L. (1987), 'Caring about and caring for the psychosocial needs of patients', *J. Fam. Pract.*, **24**(5), 461–3.

Silverman, J., Kurtz, S., and Draper, J. (1998), *Skills for communicating with patients*, Radcliffe Medical Press, Abingdon.

Silverman, J., Kurtz, S. M., and Draper, J. (1996), 'The Calgary-Cambridge approach to communication skills teaching 1: agenda-led outcome-based analysis of the consultation', *Edu. Gen. Prac.*, **7**, 288–99.

Simpson, M., Buckman, R., Stewart, M., Maguire, P., Lipkin, M., Novack, D., and Till, J. (1991), 'Doctor–patient communication: the Toronto consensus statement', *BMJ*, **303**(6814), 1385–7.

Skelton, J. R. and Hobbs, F. D. (1999), 'Descriptive study of cooperative language in primary care consultations by male and female doctors', *BMJ*, **318**(7183), 576–9.

Skelton, J. R., Kai, J., and Loudon, R. F. (2001), 'Cross-cultural communication in medicine: questions for educators', *Med. Educ.*, **35**(3), 257–61.

Smith, D. and Smith, S. J. (1999). 'Evaluating Chinese hospice care', *Health Commun.*, **11**, 226.

Smith, D., Garko, M., Bennett, K., Irwin, H., and Schofield, T. (1994), 'Patient preferences for delegation and participation: Cross-national support for mutuality', *Aus. J. Commun.*, **21**(2), 86–108.

Smith, R. (1998), 'All changed, changed utterly. British medicine will be transformed by the Bristol case', *BMJ*, **316**(7149), 1917–18.

Spence, J. (1960), *The purpose and practice of medicine*, Oxford University Press, London.

Stevenson, F. A., Barry, C. A., Britten, N., Barber, N., and Bradley, C. P. (2000), 'Doctor–patient communication about drugs: the evidence for shared decision making', *Soc. Sci. Med.*, **50**(6), 829–40.

Stewart, M. *et al.* (1995), *Patient-centered medicine: transforming the clinical method*, Sage, Thousand Oaks.

Stewart, M. A. (1995), 'Effective physician–patient communication and health outcomes: a review', *CMAJ*, **152**(9), 1423–33.

Stimson, G. V. and Webb, B. (1975), *Going to see the doctor*, Routledge and Kegan Paul, London.

Stott, N. C. and Davis, R. H. (1979), 'The exceptional potential in each primary care consultation', *J. R. Coll. Gen. Pract.*, **29**(201), 201–5.

Stott, N. C. and Pill, R. M. (1990), 'Advise yes, dictate no'. Patients' views on health promotion in the consultation', *Fam. Pract.*, **7**(2), 125–31.

Streiner, D. and Norman, G. (1995), *Health measurement scales: a practical guide to their development and use*, Oxford University Press, Oxford.

Tate, P., Foulkes, J., Neighbour, R., Campion, P., and Field, S. (1999), 'Assessing physicians' interpersonal skills via videotaped encounters: a new approach for the Royal College of General Practitioners Membership examination', *J. Health Commun.*, **4** (2), 143–52.

Towle, A. and Godolphin, W. (1999), 'Framework for teaching and learning informed shared decision making', *BMJ*, **319**(7212), 766–71.

Tuckett, D. (1976), *An introduction to medical sociology*, Tavistock, London.

Tuckett, D., Boulton, M., Olson, C., and Williams, A. (1985), *Meetings between experts: an approach to sharing medical ideas in medical consultations*, Tavistock, London.

Wallston, B. D. and Wallston, K. A. (1978), 'Locus of control and health: a review of the literature', *Health Educ. Monogr*, **6** (2), 107–17.

Williams, S., Weinman, J., Dale, J., and Newman, S. (1995), 'Patient expectations: what do primary care patients want from the GP and how far does meeting expectations affect patient satisfaction?', *Fam. Pract.*, **12**(2), 193–201.

Winefield, H. R., Murrell, T. G., and Clifford, J. (1995), 'Process and outcomes in general practice consultations: problems in defining high quality care', *Soc. Sci. Med.*, **41**(7), 969–75.

Index